I know that most men,

including those at ease with problems

of the greatest complexity, can seldom accept

even the simplest and most obvious truth

if it would oblige them to admit the falsity

of conclusions which they have delighted in

explaining to colleagues, proudly taught to others,

and which they have woven, thread by thread,

into the fabric of their lives.

Leo Tolstoy

"*A succinct summary of the gaping holes in the official view of AIDS, this book has become an underground classic. Christine Maggiore, whose own HIV positive diagnosis didn't stop her from disobeying the authorities and giving birth to a healthy child, challenges all the politically correct opinions about the health crisis. A straightforward, jargon-free little book that provides volumes of highly explosive intellectual ammunition in its brief pages.*"

IAN YOUNG • Author, *The Stonewall Experiment: A Gay Psychohistory*

"*Clear, concise and completely accurate, Christine Maggiore's powerful little book is highly recommended reading for anyone who has ever had the slightest doubt about any aspect of the 'global AIDS pandemic,' and is absolutely compulsory reading for those few who never have.*"

HARVEY BIALY, PhD • Editor at large, *Nature Biotechnology*

"*This splendid book is a perfect text for provoking university students. It requires them to think critically about sexuality and public health, obliging them to scrutinize the unscientific dogmas churned out by the AIDS orthodoxy. Maggiore's book should be required reading for all undergraduates.*"

CHARLES GESHEKTER, PhD • Department of History,
California State University, Chico

"*This book exposes the many incongruencies in conventional wisdom and establishes why we must question how AIDS research and treatment are currently conducted. The paradox of the search for an AIDS cure is that the thing most needed—open debate and scientific exchange—is the thing most feared by the AIDS establishment.*"

BOB GUCCIONE, Jr. • Editor and publisher, *Gear* magazine

"*Until recently, I was a physician at the University of Alabama at Birmingham, the number-one funded AIDS research center in the country. Before January of 1998, my knowledge of AIDS was typical; I knew that HIV caused AIDS because that's what the textbooks said. I had no reason to think otherwise and never knew or cared that anybody thought differently. I ordered this book on a whim, but once I started reading it, I didn't stop until I hit the back cover.*

"*I used to think that medical research wasn't politically directed and financially motivated, and that pharmaceutical companies wouldn't compromise patient well-being for a profit. I used to think the FDA was there to protect the American public. Now I know better. Now I tell the story of AIDS to anyone who will listen.*"

ROB HODSON, MD • Former professor of anesthesiology,
University of Alabama, Birmingham

"Most AIDS information books are about death; this one is about life. I can think of no higher recommendation. If you read one single book on AIDS, make it this one."

CELIA FARBER • Author, *SPIN* magazine, AIDS: Words from the Front

"I believe it is vital that the questions raised by this book be made known to the public. Apparently, only public demand can force an unbiased and thorough reevaluation of the cause(s) of AIDS and what might constitute an actual treatment. That the scientific and medical communities are touting the toxin AZT as a treatment for AIDS is unconscionable."

PAUL HEDLUND, Esq. • Who's Who in American Law, Who's Who in the World, Bar Register of Preeminent Lawyers

"I have been studying all sides of the HIV/AIDS discussion for 15 years and I can tell you that this little book captures all the important points with clarity and force."

DAVID RASNICK, PhD • Designer of protease inhibitors

"Nobody has to die of AIDS. This excellent book bravely and boldly spits in the eye of tradition. Instead of supposition, Christine provides facts—political facts, medical facts, nutritional facts—and she is right on target. Education is power. It will also give you back the life that fear threatens to steal from you."

BOB L. OWEN, PhD, DSc • Author, *Roger's Recovery from AIDS*

"Why have we unquestionably believed everything the government has told us about AIDS? Why have we not asked these questions before? A must-read for everyone if we are ever to uncover the truth about AIDS!"

Dr. LOIS LEE • Founder, Children of the Night, Recipient of the 1984 President's Volunteer Action Award

"AIDS is a cruel deception that is maintained because so many people are making money from it. Take away this money and the entire system of mythology will collapse. This single, portable book explains the HIV-causes-AIDS swindle in simple, concise language that anyone can understand."

CHARLES THOMAS, PhD • Former chair of the Cell Biology Department, Scripps Research Institute

"This short book will change your view of AIDS and the American medical establishment forever. Christine Maggiore deserves the thanks of honest people everywhere because she is doing nothing less than saving lives."

JON RAPPOPORT • Author, *AIDS Inc.*

First Printing 1996
Second Printing 1996, revised
Third Printing 1997, revised
Fourth Printing 2000, revised
Printed in the United States of America

Maggiore, Christine

What If Everything You Thought You Knew About AIDS Was Wrong?
Fourth edition, revised

ISBN 0-9674153-0-6: $10.95

Published by

The American Foundation for AIDS Alternatives
11684 Ventura Boulevard • Studio City, CA 91604

Cover design by Dennis Potokar
Graphic design by David Pasquarelli
Photograph of the author by Doug Piburn
Photograph of the author with son by Cindy Beal

What if everything you thought you knew about AIDS was wrong?

CHRISTINE MAGGIORE

FOURTH EDITION REVISED

This book is dedicated to the

memory of those who died without hope,

and to the future of those who may

live without fear.

Special Thanks

To my father Robert Maggiore who taught me to question authority and stand up for what's right; to my mother Evelyn Maggiore who, during my four years of devotion to this work has never once asked when I'm going to get a real job; to Bob Leppo for contributions of unparalleled generosity and lots of practical wisdom; to David Pasquarelli for superb graphic design and art direction and endless patience; to Paul Philpott for brilliant observations, hours of amusement, and tips on the best micro-brews; to Charles Geshekter, Rex Poindexter, and Carl Strygg for insightful editorial contributions; to David Crowe and Matt Irwin for sending volumes of references my way; to Christine Johnson for research on HIV tests; to Peter Duesberg for tremendous courage, sacrifice and perseverance; to Dave Rasnick for always being everywhere he's needed; to Kary Mullis for outspoken, unfaltering honesty; to Jon Rappoport for the encouragement to begin; to Celia Farber for valiant and eloquent AIDS reporting; to Jerry Terranova for creating Praxis/Cure Now and a safe place for questioning; to Esai Morales for consistent moral and fiscal support; to HEAL New York's Michael Ellner, Frank Buianouckas, Tom Di Ferdinando and Ed Lieb for inspiration and the opportunity to do my part; to website maestros Michael Davis and Rhett Topham; to the awesome Alive & Well Los Angeles crew Laura Ballegeer, Gary Cifra, Erik Dahlgren, Gregg Drolette, Kim Freitas, the ever enthusiastic Rodney Knoll, and Lou Rosenblate for their time, energy and friendship; to Arlen Bessey and Keith Relkin for helping make the first, second, and third edition books; to open-minded readers willing to explore new ideas; and to all the wonderful people this work has brought my way: you make every sacrifice and effort worthwhile.

Eternal appreciation to my guardian angel Garrett Sanders whose brief and amazing earthly presence spun me in the opposite direction of victimhood.

And the most special thanks of all to my future husband, partner in all that matters, and absolute best friend Robin Scovill, and our miraculous little Charles Dexter who fill my days with so much love, joy—and laundry.

Message from the Author

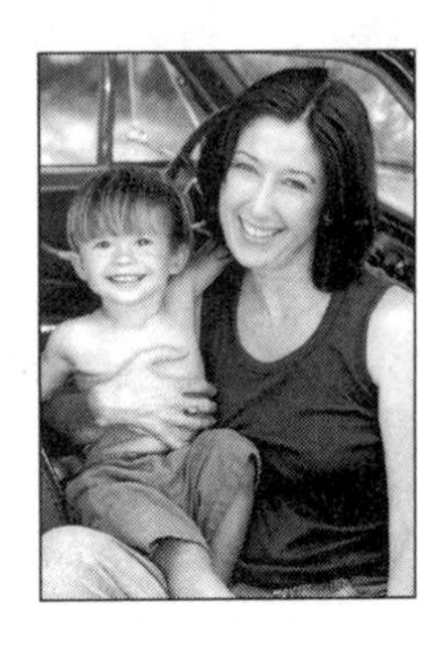

This book is actually something I never intended to write about a subject that I never imagined would touch my life. I hope you will read it with an open mind. It is a report in progress from a journey that began in 1992, when I took what is commonly referred to as an AIDS test. I had no symptoms of illness, no particular risks or fears, just a new doctor who insisted that the test should be part of a routine medical exam. My visit turned from routine to life-altering when the test came back positive.

I was referred to an AIDS specialist who declared that my test was not positive—not enough to be considered conclusive, anyway. He had me take it over again and, at the same time, ordered lab work on everything from my cholesterol level to my T cell count. I left his office frightened and confused but hopeful, and spent the days before my next appointment alternating between frantic affirmations of wellness and bottomless despair.

The result of the second test was indisputably positive. According to the specialist, my progression from somewhat positive to really positive indicated a recent infection, even though the concept of a new infection conflicted with the circumstances of my life.

He told me that I was exceptionally healthy, that I was fortunate to have detected the condition early, but that there was nothing I could do to prevent devastating disease and an eventual death from AIDS. He warned me against wasting money on vitamins and other foolish attempts to save my immune system, advising that I simply wait to become sick and then take AZT, a drug with severe side effects that would make me sicker. I was given five to seven years to live. I went directly from his office to a health food store. The following day, I began a search for a new AIDS specialist.

Life as I had lived, planned and hoped came to a grinding halt. I lost interest in my business, I dropped out of the university program I had been attending, and I bought myself a wedding ring to ward off potential suitors. Wanting to keep my tragedy a secret, I stopped spending time with my family and all but a few close friends. Instead, I attended AIDS seminars and joined a support group for HIV positive women where once a week, we were encouraged to compare notes on our fears and frustrations, mention any potential symptoms, and cry about the lousy deal we'd all been handed.

I was drafted into AIDS activism when a friend tried, in my honor, to volunteer her time at AIDS Project Los Angeles (APLA) and was turned away. Incensed that a warm, intelligent person with the sincerest of motivations would be rejected, I made my thoughts known to the men in charge. In the middle of my tirade, I was asked to join their public speaker's bureau. Almost immediately,

I was touring local high schools and colleges as the person that HIV should have never happened to. APLA booked me for a year's worth of engagements before I'd even finished their training course. I made the audiences laugh, cry, and scared—I appeared as the embodiment of the slogan that everyone is at risk for AIDS. My suggestions to brighten up the women's HIV support group at LA Shanti turned into an invitation to speak for that organization, which led to a position on the board of yet another AIDS group, Women At Risk.

A year or so into my diagnosis and public service, and after interviewing half a dozen AIDS doctors whose recommendations ranged from immediate drug therapy to world travel, I found an anomaly among AIDS specialists—a doctor who didn't routinely fill people with toxic pharmaceuticals and lethal predictions. She treated me as an individual rather than an impending statistic, and in doing so noticed my good health. She told me that I didn't fit the profile of an AIDS patient, and urged me to take another test. Afraid to raise my hopes, at first I refused. When I finally found the courage to retest, the result was inconclusive. Further testing produced a series of unsettling, contradictory diagnoses: a positive followed by a negative and another positive.

Confused by a personal situation that defied all the rules I'd been so passionately preaching as a public speaker, I turned to the AIDS groups where I worked for help. Instead of finding answers, I found my questions were dismissed, and that persisting with my line of inquiry resulted only in meaningless explanations and the distinct impression that I was ruining morale.

My search for information led me outside the confines of the AIDS establishment and into a body of scientific, medical and epidemiological data that defied everything I had been taught about AIDS, and everything that I had been teaching others. The more I read, the more I became convinced that AIDS research had jumped on a bandwagon that was headed in the wrong direction.

Since it was clear that the information I had found, however life-affirming, was not welcome among the AIDS organizations I belonged to, I decided to start my own. In 1995, together with a few friends gathered from various support groups and other places along the way, I started an organization that shares vital facts about HIV and AIDS that are unavailable from mainstream venues. A year later, while trying to write a simple threefold brochure, the first version of this book emerged. Now in its fourth printing, there are editions in Spanish, Portuguese, and Italian—and even a bootleg version in French.

In the seven years since receiving my death sentence, I have gone from frightened victim to AIDS activist to HIV dissident to spokesperson for new views about HIV and AIDS. Although my HIV status has been decidedly positive for the past five years, I enjoy abundant good health and live without pharmaceutical treatments or fear of AIDS.

In 1996, I met a wonderful man I plan to marry as soon as I take a day off. We have a beautiful, healthy little boy who at age two, has never had so much as an ear infection and is so bright that he already speaks in complete sentences.

For most people, the surprising thing about my story is the fact that it is not unusual—I know hundreds of HIV positives who are alive and naturally well years after receiving their own dire prognoses. Contrary to popular claims, what we all have in common is not some unique genetic quality, but information that liberates us from unfounded fear and allows us to embrace our natural ability to be well. A few of their stories—just the tip of an enormous and widely ignored iceberg—are included as an appendix to this book. I believe these personal accounts supplement the referenced data, and for some readers may be more meaningful than all the biomedical and epidemiological facts.

Rather than being discouraged by my experiences with a closed-minded AIDS establishment, I am encouraged by the letters and emails that arrive daily from people whose lives have been touched by this information. I receive pictures of babies that otherwise might not have been born, thanks from grateful parents who no longer worry for their grown children, messages from once-ill and hopeless AIDS patients who have restored their health and their faith in the future, accounts from people diagnosed HIV positive who go from constant terror and feelings of tragedy to calmly making the decision that HIV won't define or limit their lives, notes from teachers grateful to learn of critical thinkers, and letters from students who feel betrayed by the AIDS campaigns that have shaped their world view. I am moved by those whose messages I can't return because they're hiding their HIV status, by urgent requests for help from expectant mothers who want to protect their babies from experimental drugs, by letters from partners who tell me that the information arrived too late for someone they loved, and by the courage people find to stand up, often alone, in their conviction to lead a long and healthy life despite what the whole world believes about HIV. These notes remind me of how grateful I am to the doctors, scientists, researchers and activists who gave me the information that turned my own positive test into a way to help others, and who continue to support my efforts today.

This book is a work in progress. I value your input and comments, and make every effort to improve each edition. Please feel free to contact me with your thoughts or suggestions.

I thank you for your willingness to consider another view of AIDS.

Foreword

*"As Leonard Cohen said, 'There's a crack in everything.
That's how the light gets in.'*

*"This little opus by Christine Maggiore is a crack of brilliant white light.
It comes brightly onto a parched plain of AIDS science gone dark in our time.
She writes clearly, for any reader, the simple truth about AIDS.
And finally, it feels like rain.*

*"You guys at the NIH and the CDC, get out your umbrellas.
And you dry dogs at Glaxo-Wellcome, find a place to hide.
Because, thank truth and beauty and all the other little quarks,
at last it feels like rain."*

Kary Mullis, PhD

1993 Nobel Laureate for the invention
of the polymerase chain reaction (PCR)

Table of Contents

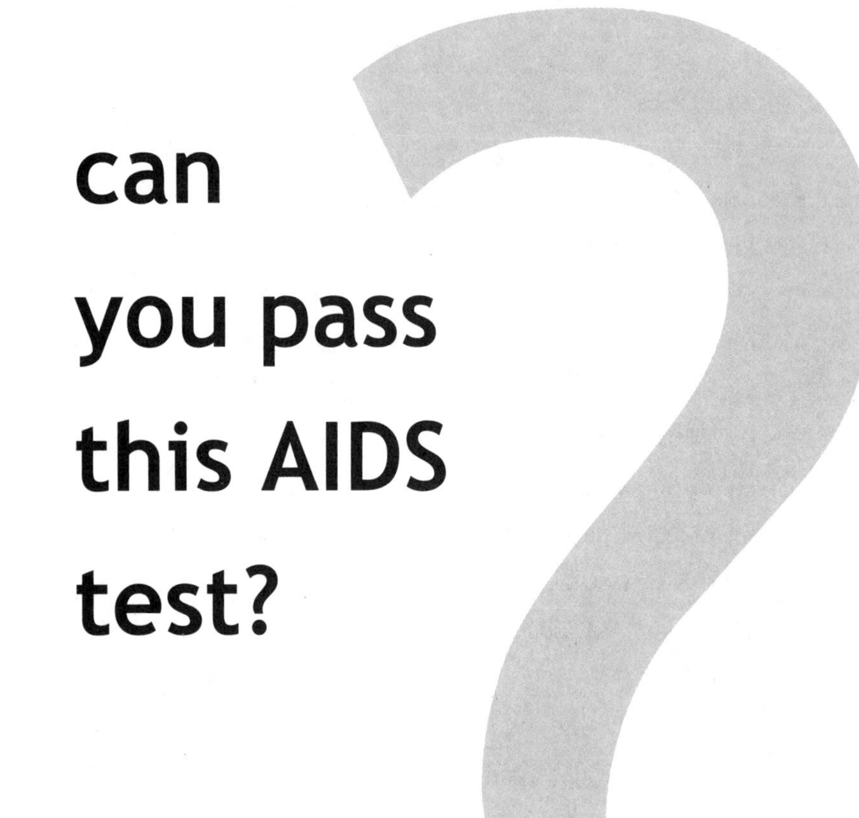

can you pass this AIDS test?

true or false?

1. AIDS is a new disease.
2. HIV is the virus that causes AIDS.
3. The "AIDS test" is extremely accurate.
4. The rate of HIV infection in America increases every year.
5. AIDS is our nation's biggest health threat.
6. AIDS is a growing risk for women, heterosexuals, and teenagers.
7. The African continent is being devastated by AIDS.
8. New AIDS drugs are responsible for recent declines in AIDS.
9. HIV causes AIDS years after infection.
10. Without medical intervention, pregnant women who test HIV positive will give their children AIDS.

All ten of these statements are

false

Surprised?

Most of our impressions about HIV and AIDS are actually based on popular ideas that have little or no basis in scientific fact.

The following pages present factual information that will change the way you think about HIV and AIDS... and possibly change your life!

1 Is AIDS a New Disease?

Contrary to popular belief, **AIDS** is not new and is not a disease. AIDS is a new name given by the Centers for Disease Control (CDC) to a collection of 29 familiar illnesses and conditions including yeast infection, herpes, diarrhea, some pneumonias, certain cancers, salmonella, and tuberculosis.[1] These illnesses are called AIDS only when they occur in a person who also has protective disease fighting proteins or **antibodies** that are thought to be associated with **HIV**.

A person is diagnosed with AIDS if they have one or more of the 29 official AIDS-defining conditions and if they also test positive for antibodies associated with HIV. In other words, pneumonia in a person who tests HIV positive is AIDS, while the same pneumonia in a person testing HIV negative is pneumonia. The clinical manifestations and symptoms of the pneumonia may be identical, but one is called AIDS while the other is just called pneumonia.

Formula for AIDS

Pneumonia	+	Positive HIV Test	=	AIDS
Pneumonia	+	Negative HIV Test	=	Pneumonia
Tuberculosis	+	Positive HIV Test	=	AIDS
Tuberculosis	+	Negative HIV Test	=	Tuberculosis

This formula creates the illusion of a perfect correlation between HIV and AIDS.

None of the 29 AIDS illnesses are new, none appear exclusively in people who test positive for HIV antibodies, and all have documented causes and treatments that are unrelated to HIV. Prior to the CDC's creation of the AIDS category, these 29 old diseases and conditions were not thought to have a single, common cause.

Although most of us associate AIDS with severe illness, on January 1, 1993, the CDC expanded the definition of AIDS to include people with a **T cell** count of 200 or less who have no illness or symptoms.[2] This new definition caused the number of AIDS cases in America to double overnight.[3] Since 1993, more than half of all new AIDS cases diagnosed each year have been among people who have no clinical symptoms or disease.[4]

AIDS: Acquired Immune Deficiency Syndrome.

Antibodies: Proteins that are manufactured by lymphocytes (a type of white blood cell) to neutralize an antigen (foreign protein) in the body. Bacteria, viruses and other microorganisms commonly contain many antigens; antibodies formed against these antigens help the body neutralize or destroy the invading microbe. Antibodies may also be formed in response to vaccines.

HIV: Human Immunodeficiency Virus; the alleged cause of AIDS.

T cell: One of the two main classes of lymphocytes. T cells play an important role in the body's immune system.

It is only through expansions of the AIDS definition that the number of new AIDS cases has grown. The definition of AIDS in America has been expanded three times since 1981. Although each addition to the definition has caused significant increases in the number of new AIDS cases, AIDS had leveled off in all risk groups by 1992 and has been declining steadily since the second quarter of 1993.

If the CDC had continued to use the first three definitions of AIDS, new American AIDS cases for 1997 would have totaled just over 10,000, making AIDS a relatively insignificant health problem. Using the 1993 definition, 21,000 new cases of AIDS were added to the year's total, and of these, more than 20,000 cases were counted among people with no symptoms or illness.[5]

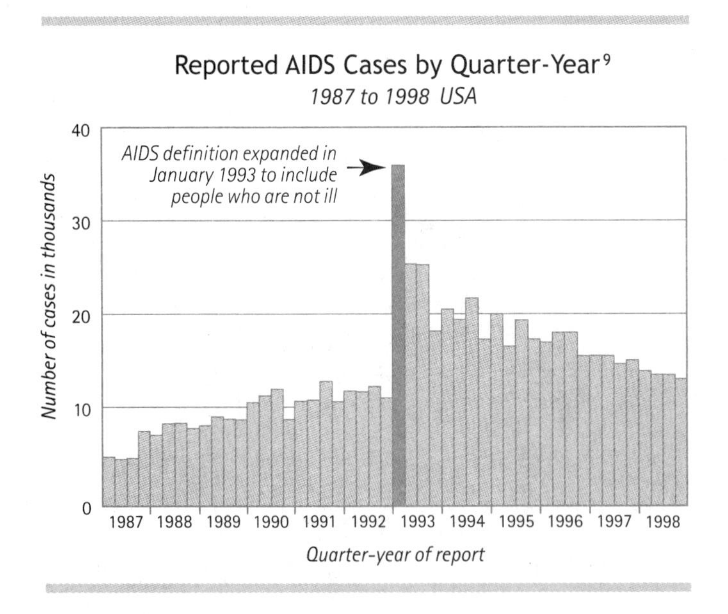

In 1998, the CDC ceased providing information on what AIDS diseases or definitions qualify people for an AIDS diagnosis each year. This means that the public will no longer know how many new AIDS cases are diagnosed in people who are not ill.[6]

Another surprising fact is that you can receive a diagnosis of AIDS without ever having an HIV test. This is referred to as a "presumptive diagnosis." According to CDC records, more than 62,000 American AIDS cases have been diagnosed with no HIV test.[7] Even though the only difference between "pneumonia" and "AIDS" is a positive HIV test, the test is not required for a diagnosis of AIDS.

Since AIDS is not a disease, and there is no single, universally accepted definition for AIDS, the conditions that are called AIDS vary from country to country. For example, Canada's Laboratory Centre for Disease Control (LCDC) does not recognize the American T cell count criteria for AIDS.[8] This means that 182,200 American AIDS patients—more than 25% of all people in the US ever diagnosed with AIDS—would not have AIDS if they were in Canada.

The World Health Organization (WHO) employs two distinctly different definitions for AIDS in Africa, neither of which conform to the criteria for American AIDS or Canadian AIDS. The diagnostic definition most commonly used in Africa does not require an HIV test, only that a patient have at least one of three major clinical symptoms (weight loss, fever and/or cough), plus one "minor sign" such as generalized itching or swollen glands.[10]

Before bringing us AIDS, the CDC attempted to sound similar alarms over relatively insignificant health matters. In 1976, after five soldiers stationed at a military base in New Jersey contracted the flu, CDC officials announced an imminent influenza epidemic. Their news releases predicted an outbreak that could wipe out as many as 500,000 Americans within a year. Congress responded to the CDC warnings by diverting millions of federal dollars into an emergency vaccine program, and following appeals from US President Gerald Ford, multitudes of concerned Americans received Swine Flu shots. However, no epidemic ever materialized and no substantiation for the notion of a life-threatening pig **virus** was ever found. Instead, more than 600 people were left paralyzed by the vaccine which also caused nearly 100 deaths.[11]

The CDC raised public concern again the next year with harrowing predictions for Legionnaire's Disease. Following massive government research efforts and relentless media reports of a new contagious disease, the form of common pneumonia dubbed "Legionnaire's" ended up taking the lives of less than 30 people nationwide. It was later discovered that 20 to 30 percent of Americans are positive for the Legionella bacteria, a common **microbe** found in water systems throughout the country.[12] The CDC's preoccupation with contagious illness contrasts with the fact that all infectious diseases combined take the lives of less than 1% of modern day Americans.[13]

AIDS in America

- AIDS is a category, not an illness.
- There are 29 familiar conditions in this category including pneumonia, yeast infections, salmonella, and certain cancers.
- None of these conditions are new.
- None of these conditions appear exclusively in people who test HIV positive; all appear among people who test HIV negative.
- All AIDS conditions have documented causes and treatments that are unrelated to HIV.

Virus: An organism comprised mainly of genetic material within a protein coat. Depending on the type of virus, the nucleic acid may be either DNA or RNA; in retroviruses, the nucleic acid is RNA. Viruses are incapable of activities typical of life such as growth, respiration and metabolism. Outside living cells, viruses are wholly inert.

Microbe: A minute form of life; a microorganism, especially one that causes disease.

2 Is HIV the Cause of AIDS?

There is no proof that HIV causes AIDS. In fact, all the epidemiological and microbiological evidence taken together conclusively demonstrates that HIV cannot cause AIDS or any other illness. The concept that AIDS is caused by a virus is not a fact, but a belief that was introduced at a 1984 press conference by Dr. Robert Gallo, a researcher employed by the National Institutes of Health (NIH).[14]

HIV is a retrovirus, a type of virus studied meticulously during two decades of federal health programs that centered around the search for a cancer virus. The idea of contagious cancer was a popular notion in the 1960s and 70s. Since retroviruses have no cell-killing mechanisms, and cancer is a condition marked by rapid cell growth, this type of virus was considered a viable candidate for the cause of cancer. However, healthy people live in harmony with an uncountable number of harmless retroviruses; some are infectious while others are **endogenous**, produced by our own **DNA**.[15] Few, if any, retroviruses have been shown to cause disease in humans.

In the 1980s when the CDC began to direct its attention to AIDS, Gallo and other cancer researchers switched their focus from cancer to the newly identified dilemma called AIDS, and the same government scientists who led the quest for a cancer virus began to search for a virus that could cause AIDS.

On April 23, 1984, Gallo called an international press conference in conjunction with the US Department of Health and Human Services (HHS). He used this forum to announce his discovery of a new retrovirus described as "the probable cause of AIDS." Although Gallo presented no evidence to support his tentative assumption, the HHS immediately characterized it as "another miracle of American medicine...the triumph of science over a dreaded disease."[16]

Later that same day, Gallo filed a patent for the antibody test now known as the "AIDS test." By the following day, *The New York Times* had turned Gallo's proposal into a certainty with front page news of "the virus that causes AIDS," and all funding for research into other possible causes of AIDS came to an abrupt halt.[17]

By announcing his **hypothesis** to the media without providing substantiating data, Gallo violated a fundamental rule of the scientific process. Researchers must first publish evidence for a hypothesis in a medical or scientific journal, and document the research or experiments that were used to construct it. Experts then examine and debate the hypothesis, and attempt to duplicate the original experiments to confirm or refute the original findings. Any new hypothesis must stand up to the scrutiny of peer review and must be verified by successful experiments before it can be considered a reasonable theory.

Endogenous: Produced from within; originating within an organ or part.

DNA: The commonly used abbreviation for deoxyribonucleic acid, the principle carrier of genetic information in almost all organisms. DNA controls a cell's activities by specifying and regulating the synthesis of enzymes and other proteins in the cell.

Hypothesis: An unproven assumption tentatively accepted as a basis for further investigation and argument.

In the case of HIV, Gallo announced an unconfirmed hypothesis to the media who reported his idea as if it were an established fact, inciting government officials to launch new public health policies based on the unsubstantiated notion of an AIDS virus. Some attribute these violations of the scientific process to the atmosphere of terror and desperation that surrounded the notion of an infectious epidemic.

The data Gallo used to construct his HIV/AIDS hypothesis were published several days after his announcement. Rather than supporting his hypothesis, this paper revealed that Gallo was unable to find HIV (actual virus) in more than half of the AIDS patients in his study.[18] While he was able to detect antibodies in most, antibodies alone are not an indication of current infection and are actually an indication of immunity from infection.

His paper also failed to provide a credible explanation as to how a retrovirus could cause AIDS. Gallo suggested that HIV worked by destroying immune cells, but 70 years of medical research had shown that retroviruses are unable to kill cells, and he offered no proof that HIV differed from other harmless retroviruses. In fact, all evidence to date conclusively demonstrates that HIV—like all retroviruses—is not **cytotoxic**.

The focus of questions about HIV quickly shifted from how it could cause AIDS to who found the now valuable viral commodity after Dr. Luc Montagnier of the Pasteur Institute in France accused Gallo of stealing his HIV sample. A congressional investigation determined that Gallo had presented fraudulent data in his original paper on HIV, and that the virus he claimed to have discovered had been sent to him by Montagnier.[19] Negotiations were conducted between the French and American governments to establish discovery and patent rights.[20] These ended in a compromise, with Montagnier and Gallo sharing credit as the codiscoverers of HIV and ownership rights to the HIV test. Montagnier has since stated that he does not believe HIV alone is capable of causing AIDS.[21]

Why HIV Cannot Cause AIDS[22]

- HIV is a retrovirus. Retroviruses are not cytotoxic; they do not kill cells.
- HIV shares the same genetic structure as all other known retroviruses. Hundreds of retroviruses are normally found in healthy human beings.
- Even if HIV could kill T cells, it only infects on average 1 in 1,000 T cells which is not enough to deplete T cells and cause AIDS.
- Most healthy people have had infections with cell-killing viruses like those that cause herpes and mononucleosis. These viruses infect millions of T cells —up to half of all immune cells—without causing T cell depletion and without causing AIDS.

Cytotoxic: Able to kill or damage cells.

Since 1984, more than 100,000 papers have been published on HIV. None of these papers, singly or collectively, has been able to reasonably demonstrate or effectively prove that HIV causes AIDS. Although Gallo claimed that HIV caused AIDS by destroying the T cells of the immune system, 20 years of cancer research confirmed that retroviruses are not cytotoxic. In fact, there is still no evidence in the scientific literature demonstrating that HIV is able to destroy T cells, directly or indirectly.

Comparing HIV to Varicella Zoster Virus (VZV), the known cause of chicken pox, highlights some of the ways in which HIV defies rules of science and logic.

HIV Bends the Rules of Science

VZV = Chicken Pox	HIV = AIDS?
Same symptoms in all cases	Different symptoms depending on risk group
Natural VZV antibodies, in the absence of virus, indicate life-long immunity	Natural HIV antibodies, in the absence of virus, said to indicate or predict AIDS
VZV (actual virus) is readily found in all cases of chicken pox	HIV (actual virus) is rarely found in cases of AIDS
VZV (actual virus) is readily found in high concentrations in affected tissues of ill patients	HIV (actual virus) is rarely found and only in low concentrations in T cells of ill patients
VZV replication kills cells	HIV replication does not kill cells
Most severe symptoms appear days or weeks after infection and before antibody immunity (VZV+)	AIDS symptoms said to occur years after infection and only after antibody immunity (HIV+)

HIV is the only virus that is said to cause a group of diseases caused by other viruses and bacteria rather than causing its own disease. AIDS experts also say that HIV is able to cause cell depletion—loss of immune cells—at the same time it causes cell proliferation or cancer.

Although more research money has been spent on HIV than on the combined total of all other viruses studied in medical history, there is no scientific evidence validating the hypothesis that HIV is the cause of AIDS, or that AIDS has a viral cause. A good hypothesis is defined by its ability to solve problems and mysteries, make accurate predictions and produce results. The HIV hypothesis has failed to meet any of these criteria.

Hundreds of scientists around the world are now requesting an official reevaluation of the HIV hypothesis. For more information on their efforts, refer to *The Group for the Scientific Reappraisal of the HIV/AIDS Hypothesis* on page 76.

3 Is the "AIDS Test" Accurate?

Many people are surprised to learn that there is no such thing as a test for AIDS. The tests popularly referred to as "AIDS tests" do not identify or diagnose AIDS and cannot detect HIV, the virus claimed to cause AIDS. The ELISA and Western Blot tests commonly used to diagnose HIV infection detect only interactions between proteins and antibodies thought to be specific for HIV—they do not detect HIV itself. And contrary to popular belief, newer "viral load" tests do not measure levels of actual virus in the blood.

All HIV antibody tests are highly inaccurate. One reason for the tests' tremendous inaccuracy is that a variety of viruses, bacteria and other **antigens** can cause the immune system to make antibodies that also react with HIV. When the antibodies produced in response to these other infections and antigens react with HIV proteins, a positive result is registered. Many antibodies found in normal, healthy, HIV-free people can cause a positive reading on HIV antibody tests.[23] Since the antibody production generated by a number of common viral infections can continue for years after the immune system has defeated a virus—and even for an entire lifetime—people never exposed to HIV can have consistent **false positive** reactions on HIV tests for years or for their entire lives.

The accuracy of an antibody test can be established only by verifying that positive results are found in people who actually have the virus. This standard for determining accuracy was not met in 1984 when the HIV antibody test was first created. Instead, to this day, positive ELISAs are verified by a second antibody test of unknown accuracy, the HIV Western Blot. Since the accuracy for HIV antibody tests has never been properly established, it is not possible to claim that a positive test indicates a current, active HIV infection or even to know what it may indicate.[24] In one study that investigated positive results confirmed by Western Blot, 80 people with two positive ELISAs that were "verified" by a positive Western Blot tested negative on their next Western Blot.[25]

Antibodies produced in response to simple infections like a cold or the flu can cause a positive reaction on an HIV antibody test. A flu shot and other immunizations can also create positive HIV ELISA and Western Blot results. Having or having had herpes or hepatitis may produce a positive test, as can vaccination for hepatitis B. Exposure to microbes such as those that cause tuberculosis and malaria commonly cause false positive results, as do the presence of tapeworms and other parasites. Conditions such as alcoholism or liver disease and blood that is altered through drug use may elicit the production of antibodies that react on HIV antibody tests. Pregnancy and prior pregnancy can also cause a positive response. The antibodies produced to act against

Antigen: A substance that can trigger an immune response, resulting in the production of antibodies as part of the body's defense system against infection and disease. Many antigens are foreign proteins (those not found naturally in the body); they include microorganisms, toxins, and tissues from another person used in organ transplantation. Antigen stands for ANTIbody GENerating.

False positive: Indicates infection where none exists.

infection with mycobacterium and yeast, infections which are found in 90% of AIDS patients, cause false positive HIV test results.[26] In one study, 13% of Amazonian Indians who do not have AIDS and who have no contact with people outside their own tribe tested HIV positive.[26] In another report, 50% of blood samples from healthy dogs reacted positively on HIV antibody tests.[27]

Prior to the notion that HIV causes AIDS, viral antibodies were considered a normal, healthy response to infection and an indication of immunity. Antibodies alone were not used to diagnose disease or predict illness. Before HIV, only ELISA and Western Blot tests that had been shown to correspond with the finding of actual virus were used to diagnose viral infections. There is no credible scientific evidence to suggest that these rules should be disregarded to accommodate HIV.

In addition to being inaccurate, HIV antibody tests are not standardized. This means that there is no nationally or internationally accepted criteria for what constitutes a positive result. Standards also vary from lab to lab within the same country or state, and can even differ from day to day at the same lab.[28] As HIV test kit manufacturers acknowledge, "At present there is no recognized standard for establishing the presence or absence of antibodies to HIV-1 and HIV-2 in human blood."[29]

The following chart illustrates just some of the varying criteria for what is considered a positive HIV Western Blot, and shows how someone could actually switch from positive to negative simply by changing countries. The differing standards for positive HIV tests are not limited to the locations and agencies mentioned here—criteria vary from lab to lab and results are open to interpretation. An inconclusive test can become positive or negative based on an individual's sexual preference, health history, zip code or other survey data.

Varying Criteria for a Positive HIV Western Blot[30]

Gene	Proteins	AFRICA	AUSTRALIA	UNITED KINGDOM	USA CDC 1	USA CDC 2	USA FDA	USA RED CROSS
ENV gene	p160 p120 p41	ANY TWO	ONE OR MORE	ONE OR MORE	p120/ p160* AND p41	p120/ p160* OR p41	ONE OR MORE	ONE OR MORE
POL gene	p68 p53 p32	OPTIONAL	ANY THREE	p31**			p32	ANY ONE
GAG gene	p55 p40 p24			p24		p24	p24	ANY ONE

* The CDC regards p120 and p160 as a single unit—if antibodies to one show up, the others are automatically considered to be present

** Used instead of p32 in the United Kingdom

The various proteins used in HIV Western Blot tests are arranged into bands that are divided into three sections. These three sections are represented by the abbreviations ENV, POL and GAG. Proteins in the ENV section correspond to the outer membrane or "envelope" of a virus; POL refers to proteins common to all retroviruses which include polymerase and other enzymes; GAG stands for "group specific antigen" and includes proteins that form the inner core of a virus. The protein bands in each section are indicated by the letter "p" and are followed by a number which describes the molecular weight of that protein measured in daltons. For example, p160 is an ENV protein that weighs 160 daltons.

It is important to note that none of the proteins used in HIV antibody tests are particular to HIV, and none of the antigens said to be specific to HIV are found only in persons who test HIV positive. In fact, many people diagnosed HIV positive do not have these "HIV antigens" in their blood.

As mentioned previously, newer HIV "viral load" tests do not isolate or measure actual virus. The tests' manufacturers clearly state that viral load "is not intended to be used as a screening test for HIV or as a diagnostic test to confirm the presence of HIV infection."[31] In fact, viral load tests have not been approved by the FDA for diagnostic purposes and have not been verified by virus isolation. For more information on viral load tests, please see *What's Up With Viral Load?* on page 36. Of course, the most outstanding problem with any HIV test is that HIV has never been demonstrated to cause AIDS.

Should You Bet Your Life on an HIV Test?

"The only way to distinguish between real reactions and cross-reactions is to use HIV isolation. All claims of HIV isolation are based on a set of phenomena detected in tissue culture, none of which are isolation and none of which are even specific for retroviruses...We don't know how many positive tests occur in the absence of HIV infection. There is no specificity of the HIV antibody tests for HIV infection."

Bio/Technology Journal, 11:696-707, 1993

"The HIV antibody tests do not detect a virus. They test for any antibodies that react with an assortment of proteins experts claim are specific to HIV. The fact is that an antibody test, even if repeated and found positive a thousand times, does not prove the presence of viral infection."

Val Turner, MD, *Continuum* magazine, Vol 3 No 5, 1996

"HIV tests are notoriously unreliable in Africa. A 1994 study published in the *Journal of Infectious Diseases* concluded that HIV tests were useless in central Africa, where the microbes responsible for tuberculosis, malaria and leprosy were so prevalent that they registered over 70% false positive."

Sacramento Bee, October 30, 1994

"With public health officials and politicians thrashing out who should be tested for HIV, the accuracy of the test itself has been nearly ignored. A study last month by Congress' Office of Technology Assessment found that HIV tests can be very inaccurate indeed. For groups at very low risk—people who don't use IV drugs or have sex with gay or bisexual men—9 in 10 positive findings are called false positives, indicating infection where none exists."

US News & World Report, November 23, 1987

"People who receive gamma globulin shots for chicken pox, measles and hepatitis could test positive for HIV even if they've never been infected. The Food and Drug Administration says that a positive test could be caused by antibodies found in most of America's supply of gamma globulin. Gamma globulin is made from blood collected from thousands of donors and is routinely given to millions of people each year as temporary protection against many infectious diseases. Dr. Thomas Zuck of the FDA's Blood and Blood Products Division says the government didn't release the information because 'we thought it would do more harm than good.'"

USA Today, October 2, 1987

"Two weeks ago, a 3-year-old child in Winston Salem, North Carolina, was struck by a car and rushed to a nearby hospital. Because the child's skull had been broken and there was a blood spill, the hospital performed an HIV test. As the traumatized mother was sitting at her child's bedside, a doctor came in and told her the child was HIV-positive. Both parents are negative. The doctor told the mother that she needed to launch an investigation into her entire family and circle of friends because this child had been sexually abused. There was no other way, the doctor said, that the child could be positive. A few days later, the mother demanded a second test. It came back negative. The hospital held a press conference where a remarkable admission was made. In her effort to clear the hospital of any wrongdoing, a hospital spokesperson announced that 'these HIV tests are not reliable; a lot of factors can skew the tests, like fever or pregnancy. Everybody knows that.'"

Celia Farber, *Impression Magazine*, June 21, 1999

"A Vancouver woman is suing St. Paul's Hospital and several doctors because she was diagnosed as carrying the AIDS virus, when in fact she wasn't. In a BC Supreme Court writ, Lisa Lebed claims when she was admitted to the hospital in late 1995 to give birth to a daughter, a blood sample was taken without her consent. It revealed she was HIV positive, so she gave up the baby girl for adoption and decided to have a tubal ligation. A year and a half later, while undergoing AIDS treatment, she found out she was not HIV positive. The explanation she was given was a lab error. She says because of the negligence of the hospital, she's now sterile and has lost a daughter."

Woman Sues St. Paul's, CKNW Radio 98, June 10, 1999

Factors Known to Cause Positive Results on HIV Antibody Tests [32]

Acute viral infections, DNA viral infections[13c,40c,43c,48c,53c,59c]

Administration of human immunoglobulin preparations pooled before 1985[10c]

Alcoholic hepatitis/alcoholic liver disease[10c,13c,32c,40c,43c,48c,49c,53c]

Alpha interferon therapy in hemodialysis patients[54c]

Antibodies with a high affinity for polystyrene (used in the test kits)[3c,40c,62c]

Anti-carbohydrate antibodies[13c,19c,52c]

Anti-collagen antibodies (found in gay men, haemophiliacs, Africans of both sexes and people with leprosy)[31c]

Anti-Hbc IgM[48c]

Anti-hepatitis A IgM (antibody)[48c]

Anti-lymphocyte antibodies[31c,56c]

Anti-microsomal antibodies[34c]

Anti-mitochondrial antibodies[13c,48c]

Anti-nuclear antibodies[13c,48c,53c]

Anti-parietal cell antibody[48c]

Anti-smooth muscle antibody[48c]

Autoimmune diseases (systemic lupus erythematosus, scleroderma, connective tissue disease, dermatomyositis)[10c,29c,40c,43c,44c,49c]

Blood transfusions[13c,36c,41c,43c,49c,63c]

Epstein-Barr virus[37c]

False positives on other tests, including RPR (rapid plasma reagent) test for syphilis[10c,17c,33c,48c,49c]

Flu[36c]

Flu vaccination[3c,11c,13c,20c,30c,43c]

Globulins produced during polyclonal gammopathies (in AIDS risk groups)[10c,13c,48c]

Hemolyzed serum (blood where hemoglobin is separated from the red cells)[49c]

Hematologic malignant disorders/lymphoma[9c,13c,43c,48c,53c]

Hemophilia[10c,49c]

Heat-treated specimens[24c,48c,49c,51c,57c]

Hemodialysis/renal failure[10c,16c,41c,49c,56c]

Hepatitis[54c]

Hepatitis B vaccination[21c,28c,40c,43c]

Herpes simplex I and II[11c,27c]

High levels of circulating immune complexes[6c,33c]

HLA antibodies (to Class I and II leukocyte antigens)[7c,10c,13c,43c,46c,48c,49c,53c,63c]

Hyperbilirubinemia[10c,13c]

Hypergammaglobulinemia (high levels of antibodies)[33c,40c]

Leprosy[2c,25c]

Lipemic serum (blood with high levels of fat or lipids)[49c]

Malaria[6c,12c]

Malignant neoplasms (cancers)[40c]

Multiple myeloma[10c,43c,53c]

Mycobacterium avium[25c]

Naturally-occurring antibodies[5c,19c]

Normal human ribonucleoproteins[13c,48c]

Organ transplantation[1c,36c]

Other retroviruses[8c,13c,14c,48c,55c]

Passive immunization: receipt of gamma globulin or immune globulin (as prophylaxis against infection which contains antibodies) [4c,13c,18c,22c,26c,42c,43c,60c]

Poorly-understood cross reactions in healthy individuals[10c]

Pregnancy in multiparous women[13c,36c,43c,53c,58c]

Primary biliary cirrhosis[13c,43c,48c,53c]

Primary sclerosing cholangitis[48c,53c]

Proteins on the filter paper[13c]

Q-fever with associated hepatitis[61c]

Recent viral infection or exposure to viral vaccines[11c]

Receptive anal sex[39c,64c]

Renal (kidney) failure[13c,23c,48c]

Renal transplantation[9c,13c,35c,48c,56c]

Rheumatoid arthritis[36c]

Serum-positive for rheumatoid factor, anti-nuclear antibody (both found in rheumatoid arthritis and other autoantibodies)[14c,53c,62c]

Stevens-Johnson syndrome[9c,13c,48c]

"Sticky" blood (in Africans)[34c,38c,40c]

Systemic lupus erythematosus[15c,23c]

Tetanus vaccination[40c]

Tuberculosis[25c]

T-cell leukocyte antigen antibodies[13c,48c]

Upper respiratory tract infection (cold or flu)[11c]

Visceral leishmaniasis[45c]

4 Is the Rate of HIV Increasing?

HIV is not on the rise. According to the most recent CDC estimates, the number of HIV positive Americans has not increased once since the HIV test was introduced into general use in 1985.

In 1986, the CDC began promoting the estimate that 1 million to 1.5 million Americans were HIV positive.[33] Media and AIDS organizations employed this figure to make the disturbing claim that one in every 250 people in the nation was infected with HIV. Four years later, official estimates were lowered to between 800,000 and 1.2 million, and in 1995, following an investigation by *NBC Nightly News*, the CDC again decreased their official estimate to between 650,000 and 900,000, a figure still promoted today.[33,34]

While the number of HIV positives has failed to grow, it is important to note that rates of venereal diseases such as chlamydia, genital herpes, gonorrhea and syphilis have increased throughout most of the AIDS epidemic and far surpass cases of AIDS. These numbers contradict the idea that "safe sex" has prevented HIV from spreading.

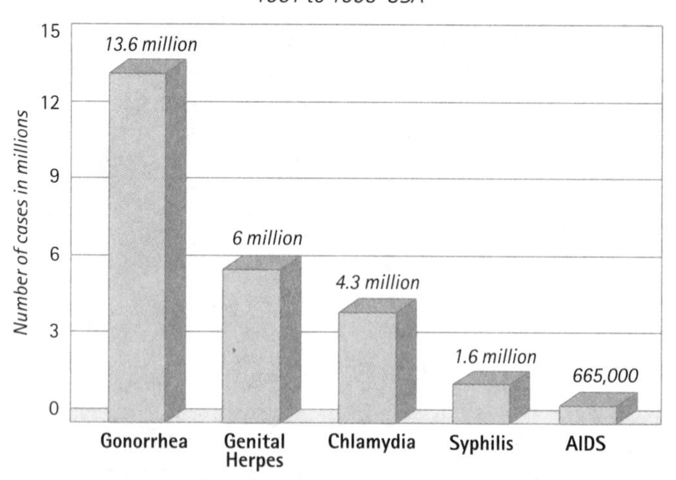

5 Is AIDS Our Biggest Health Threat?

In 1998, deaths in Americans with AIDS reached 410,800. This is the total for the entire time known as the AIDS epidemic, a period which spans nearly two decades.[36] Included in this total are deaths from any cause at all—accidents, noncontagious illnesses, drug side effects, etc.—in people diagnosed with AIDS.[37]

Without dismissing AIDS deaths or the profound suffering of AIDS patients and their loved ones, it is important to give this total some comparative perspective: Over 400,000 Americans die each year of cancer, and there are more than 700,000 annual deaths in this country from cardiovascular disease.[38]

During the period known as the AIDS epidemic, 14 million people died of heart disease—13.5 million more than have ever died of AIDS—while 9 million succumbed to cancer, which is 8.5 million more than those counted for AIDS. From 1981 to 1998, car accidents killed over 800,000 Americans—almost twice as many as have ever died of AIDS. Suicides during the AIDS epidemic surpass AIDS fatalities by more than 100,000.[38] Loss of life from adverse reactions to properly prescribed and correctly taken pharmaceuticals outnumber AIDS deaths in America by more than 1.3 million.[39]

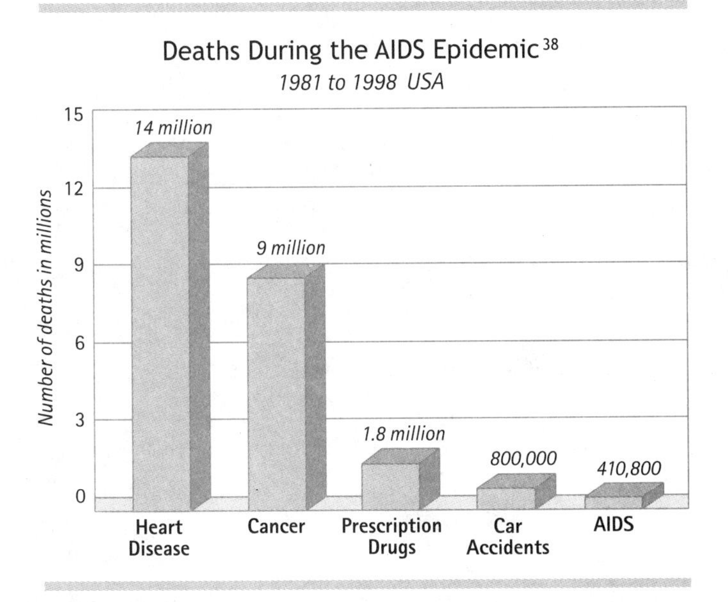

Although most people associate the word "epidemic" with AIDS, one of the last truly devastating outbreaks in history, the flu of 1918, took the lives of 20 million people worldwide in a single year.[40] After almost 20 years, diagnosed cases of AIDS throughout the world total just over 2 million, and included among these are many people who remain alive and well.[41]

So why do we think of enormous numbers whenever we think of AIDS? Unlike cancer and most other conditions, AIDS reports typically use cumulative totals. In other words, a current year's cases or fatalities are added to the sum total of all AIDS diagnoses or deaths that have ever occurred, automatically creating a larger figure and the impression that AIDS constantly rises.

Also, estimates and projections are frequently used in place of actual AIDS numbers. For example, the 1999 *United Nations AIDS Report* estimates that 2.5 million people throughout the world died of AIDS in 1998 while the November 1999 World Health Organization (WHO) *Weekly Epidemiological Record* reports that only 2.2 million people worldwide have ever received a diagnosis of AIDS.[42] The UN estimate is widely promoted while the actual WHO case count is rarely publicized.

A little reported fact is that AIDS is not among the ten leading causes of deaths for Americans. In annual death rates, AIDS lags behind motor vehicle accidents, non-vehicular accidents and adverse events, flu and pneumonia, diabetes, septicemia, Alzheimer's disease, and homicide.[43] It is often reported that AIDS is the leading cause of death among Americans aged 25 to 44. This statement inspires great fear and concern until carefully examined. Only two-tenths of one percent (0.2%) of persons in this age group die of any cause each year, and among these, deaths from AIDS represent about three one-hundredths of one percent (0.03%). However, since AIDS constitutes the leading category for fatalities at about 15% (85% of people within this age range die of other causes), it is possible to call AIDS the leading killer.[44] For more information on the use of AIDS statistics, see *Public Health, Public Relations and AIDS* on page 45.

Portraying AIDS as our biggest health threat gives AIDS funding priority over problems that affect far greater numbers of Americans. According to findings by the Institute of Medicine, NIH research expenditures in 1996 averaged $1,160 for every American who died of heart disease, $4,700 for each one who died of cancer, and more than $43,000 for every death in a person diagnosed with AIDS.[45]

False Alarms!

"By 1990, one in five heterosexuals will be dead from AIDS."

Oprah Winfrey, 1987 • *The Myth of Heterosexual AIDS*, 1990

"By 1991, HIV will have spread to between 5 and 10 million Americans."

Newsweek • November 10, 1986

"By 1991, 1 in 10 babies may be AIDS victims."

USA Today headline, 1988

"By 1996, three to five million Americans will be HIV positive and one million will be dead from AIDS."

NIAID Director Dr. Anthony Fauci • *New York Times*, January 14, 1986

"Without massive federal AIDS intervention, there may be no one left."

HHS Secretary Donna Shalala, 1993 • *Washington Times*, June 8, 1999

6 Are We All at Risk for AIDS?

It is often said that everyone is at risk for AIDS, but the actual numbers suggest otherwise. After nearly two decades, AIDS cases in this country have remained 94% confined to the originally identified risk groups.[46]

The CDC places 88% of American AIDS patients in two categories: men who have sex with men or injection drug users. Just 10% of Americans diagnosed with AIDS cite heterosexual contact as their only risk and of these, close to half (4%) mention sexual relations with users of injection drugs.

The classification of AIDS cases by risk group relies entirely on voluntary responses to CDC survey questions, a method of gathering information that is well-documented to be a source of distortion and invalidity.[47] In fact, a number of public health studies show that upon further investigation, 65% to 99% of people with AIDS who initially claim heterosexual contact as their only risk or who claim no risk at all, later acknowledge using injection drugs and/or having male homosexual relations.[48]

Although men who have sex with men is the leading risk group for an AIDS diagnosis, this information is not intended to suggest that gay male sex is a cause of AIDS, or that all men who have sex with men are at risk. There are specific health-compromising factors associated with, but that are not unique to, men who have sex with men that are known to cause acquired immune deficiency. Please see *If It's Not HIV, What Can Cause AIDS?* on page 51 for further information and clarification. It is also important to note that AIDS risk groups are limited to the six categories defined by the CDC and that the CDC accepts all survey responses regarding risks as accurate.

AIDS Cases by CDC Risk Groups[49]

AIDS by Risk Group	
Men Who Have Sex with Men	53%
Injection Drug Users	35%
Heterosexual Contact	6%
Heterosexual Contact with IDU	4%
Transfusion Recipients	1%
Hemophiliacs	1%

AIDS by Health Status	
No Illness	67%
Illness	33%

AIDS by Gender	
Male	85%
Female	15%

The risk of AIDS is also disproportionately divided among men and women in America, with 85% of cumulative AIDS cases confined to males.[50] In contrast to this fact, HIV testing conducted by the US military since 1985 reports near equal numbers of HIV positive results among male and female new recruits.[51] If HIV were the cause of AIDS, we should expect a near equal number of AIDS cases among men and women. Instead, women have never represented more than 15% of all AIDS cases nationwide.

In a contagious epidemic, healthcare professionals working among the ill usually run the highest risk of contracting a disease. During the entire AIDS epidemic however, only 25 cases of AIDS have been reported among healthcare workers who claim occupational exposure as their only risk, and none of these 25 cases have been described in the medical literature.[52] Although the CDC reports that 75% of healthcare workers are women, 23 of these 25 AIDS cases (92%) are men.[54] Also of interest is the fact that there are no emergency medical technicians, paramedics, surgeons or dentists among the 25 occupational AIDS cases reported by the CDC.[53] In comparison to AIDS, 1,000 cases of hepatitis infection are reported each year among healthcare workers who attribute their illness to occupational exposure.[54]

Questioning AIDS

- Why are 88% of Americans with AIDS confined to two risk groups?
- Why are 85% of AIDS cases in the US found among males?
- If AIDS is a widespread health risk, why has it not spread into the general population?
- Since health care workers are at high risk in any epidemic, why are there only 25 claimed cases of occupational AIDS among health care workers after nearly two decades of AIDS?
- If AIDS is a sexually transmitted disease (STD), why do cases of syphilis, chlamydia and gonorrhea far outnumber AIDS?
- Since female prostitutes are at high risk for all STDs, why are they not a risk group for AIDS?

While AIDS is often cited as the primary health risk for America's 26 million teens, according to the CDC, new AIDS cases among US teenagers in 1998 totaled 293—a drop from the previous year's total of 403.[55] The sum total for AIDS among Americans age 13 to 19 for the entire period known as the AIDS epidemic is 3,432 cases. In Canada, just two new cases of teenage AIDS were reported in 1997 while that same year Canadian teenagers accounted for half of all 4,442 new infections of gonorrhea.[56]

Pediatric AIDS is a popular topic in national news and is the focus of many multimillion dollar fund-raising efforts even though there are fewer than 400 cases of AIDS among children age five and under for each year of the AIDS epidemic.[57] Studies have shown that as many as 85% of pediatric AIDS cases in the US and Europe occur among children born to mothers who admit to using IV drugs during pregnancy.[58] New cases of pediatric AIDS—along with AIDS cases in all categories—have been decreasing steadily since 1993, and in 1998, only 10 states reported more than 10 new diagnoses of pediatric AIDS.

All AIDS cases among children age 12 and under during the AIDS epidemic total less than 8,500. Compare this to Sudden Infant Death Syndrome (SIDS) which during the same period of time has taken the lives of more than 80,000 children, all under one year of age.[59]

Actuarial calculations demonstrate that the chance of testing HIV positive following a single act of unprotected vaginal intercourse with a person outside a high risk group is one in seven million, which is less than the chance of being struck by lightning, less than the chance of dying of food poisoning at a fast-food restaurant, less than being injured in an elevator ride, and about the same odds as being killed in a traffic accident while traveling a distance of 10 miles.[60]

7 Is AIDS Devastating Africa?

According to the 1999 World Health Organization (WHO) report, the total number of actual diagnosed AIDS cases on the African continent is about equal to the total for AIDS in America even though Africa, with its 650 million people, has more than two times the population of the USA.[61] Africa is often cited as a worst case example of what could happen in America despite figures that demonstrate that 99.5% of Africans do not have AIDS, and among Africans who test HIV positive, 97% do not have AIDS.[62]

Unlike in the United States, AIDS in Africa may be diagnosed based on four clinical symptoms—fever, involuntary loss of 10% of normal body weight, persistent cough, and diarrhea—and HIV tests are not required.[63] The four clinical AIDS symptoms are identical to those associated with conditions that run rampant on the African continent such as malaria, tuberculosis, parasitic infections, the effects of malnutrition, and unsanitary drinking and bathing water. These symptoms are the result of poverty and other problems that have troubled Africa and other developing areas of the world for many decades.

What about Africa?[64]

- African AIDS is diagnosed by four clinical symptoms:
  - Diarrhea, fever, persistent cough, and weight loss of more than 10% over two months.
- HIV tests are not required for an AIDS diagnosis in Africa.
  - 99.5% of Africans do not have AIDS.
  - 97% of HIV positive Africans do not have AIDS.
- Cases of tuberculosis, malaria and measles far outnumber cases of AIDS in Africa.
- AIDS is not the leading cause of illness or death in any African nation.

The idea that AIDS originated in Africa remains popular although there has never been scientific or epidemiological evidence to substantiate this notion. News reports suggesting that HIV began in Africa as Simian Immunodeficiency Virus (SIV) are based on elaborate speculation about species-jumping viruses rather than reliable evidence.

SIV induces only flu like symptoms in some experimental laboratory monkeys and does not cause any of the 29 official AIDS-defining illnesses. Unlike HIV infection which is said to cause illness only years after exposure and despite the presence of protective antibodies, SIV will cause illness within days of infection or not at all, and wild monkeys retain SIV antibodies throughout their lives without ever becoming ill. Only monkeys in unnatural circumstances—lab animals with undeveloped immune systems who are injected with large quantities of SIV—become ill.[65]

In a recent attempt to advance the hypothesis of an SIV/HIV connection, researchers used the results of nonspecific antibody tests to claim that three chimpanzees captured in West Africa had been infected with HIV/SIV through sexual transmission. Efforts to isolate actual virus from the animals revealed that two of the three chimps had no virus, while the researchers admitted that the virus found in the one was not even closely related to HIV. Their report also failed to explain why the "infected" animals did not transmit HIV/SIV to any of the 150 other chimps living in the colony where they were kept, or why their mates and offspring did not test positive.[66]

While Africa is the frequent subject of dramatic media reports, actual numbers of diagnosed AIDS cases on the continent are relatively unremarkable. For example, 1981 through 1999 cumulative AIDS cases for South Africa, the new epicenter of AIDS, total just 12,825.[67]

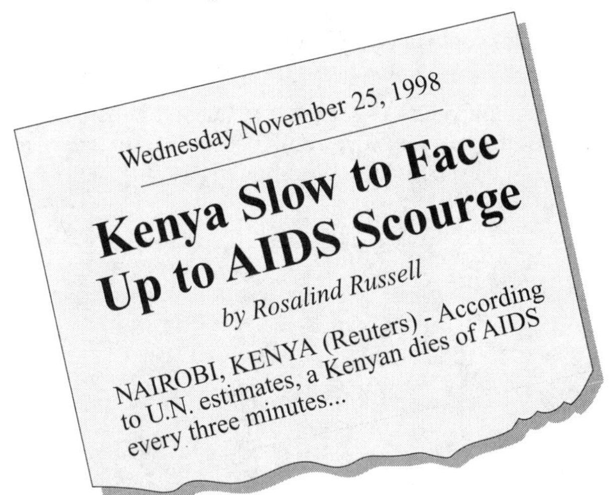

Wednesday November 25, 1998

Kenya Slow to Face Up to AIDS Scourge

by Rosalind Russell

NAIROBI, KENYA (Reuters) - According to U.N. estimates, a Kenyan dies of AIDS every three minutes...

If this news story were true...

- 480 Kenyans would die of AIDS each day;
- 175,000 Kenyans would die of AIDS every year;
- Three million Kenyans would have died of AIDS since 1981.

The fact is that in Kenya...

- There have been 81,492 diagnosed AIDS cases since 1981 and many of these are people who remain alive and well.

Unfounded estimates, rather than unprotected sex, are responsible for the alarming number of AIDS cases said to occur in Africa. United Nations' AIDS estimates were cited as the inspiration for a recent news report claiming "a Kenyan dies of AIDS every three minutes."[68] If Kenyans were dying at this rate, there would be more than twice as many dead Kenyans in just one year than have ever been actually diagnosed with AIDS in the entire period of time known as the AIDS epidemic.

In 1987, the WHO estimated there were 1 million HIV positives in Uganda, the nation then considered the epicenter of AIDS. Ten years later, WHO estimates for Uganda remained unchanged at 1 million HIV positives while the total of actual AIDS cases through 1999 are less than 55,000 in this country of more than 20 million people.[69]

AIDS is not, as many believe, Africa's primary health threat; several million cases of tuberculosis and malaria are reported each year in Africa while total AIDS cases on the continent for the entire AIDS epidemic hover just above one-half million. For example, in 1996 there were 170,000 cases of tuberculosis reported in Ethiopia and less than 850 cases of AIDS; South Africa's tuberculosis cases topped 91,000 compared to 729 diagnosed cases of AIDS. In fact, AIDS is not the leading cause of illness or death in any African country.[70]

Because of the high incidence of exposure to malaria, tuberculosis and other diseases that produce false positive results on HIV tests, many mainstream scientists question the validity of HIV testing in Africa.[71]

8 Are New Drug Treatments Responsible for Declines in AIDS?

Government officials, AIDS organizations and the media unanimously agree that the recent decline in AIDS cases and deaths is an unprecedented occurrence due to a new combination of drugs that include protease inhibitors, chemicals said to block the replication of HIV. However, a careful look behind the headlines reveals that there is no medical evidence to support these popular claims about the protease inhibitor "combo cocktails."

The declines in AIDS deaths attributed to combination therapies actually began several years before protease inhibitor drugs became available for general use.[72] Since the first protease inhibitor received Food and Drug Administration (FDA) approval in December of 1995, a more likely explanation for decreased deaths would be the change in the official AIDS definition adopted in 1993 which allows HIV positives with no symptoms or illness to be diagnosed with AIDS. Since 1993, more than half of all newly diagnosed AIDS cases are counted among people who are not sick.[73]

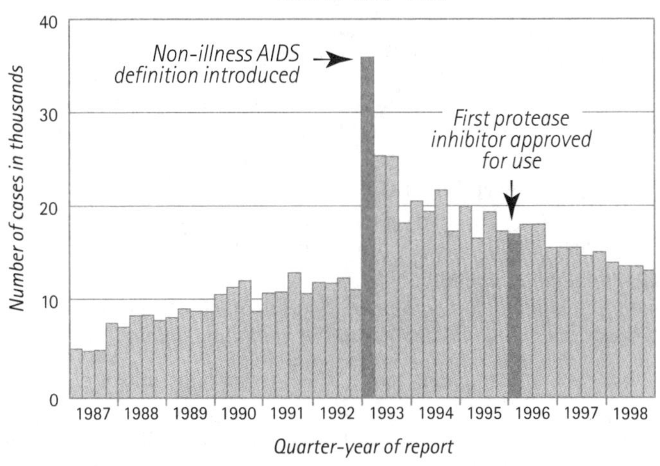

CDC data also show that decreases in AIDS cases commonly ascribed to "AIDS cocktails" preceded the introduction of the new drug treatments by three full years. According to the CDC's *HIV/AIDS Surveillance Report*, AIDS diagnoses peaked in the third quarter of 1991, increased once in the first quarter of 1993 as a result of the 1993 expanded AIDS definition, and have dropped each year since.[75]

News stories of AIDS patients who rise from their death beds to run marathons after taking the drug cocktails, are just that—stories. In science, such unverified accounts are dismissed as anecdotal, a term that comes from the Greek word *anekdotos*, meaning unpublished. None of the anecdotal tales of recoveries attributed to new drug combinations have been substantiated by controlled studies published in peer-reviewed medical journals, a fact acknowledged in the fine print of pharmaceutical advertisements:

- *"At this time there is no evidence that Ziagen will help you live longer or have fewer of the medical problems associated with HIV or AIDS."*
- *"It is not yet known whether Crixivan will extend your life or reduce your chances of getting other illnesses associated with HIV."*
- *"At present, there are no results from controlled clinical trials evaluating the effects of Viramune [on] the incidence of opportunistic infections or survival."*
- *"There have been no clinical trials conducted with Combivir."*[76]

Incomplete and inconclusive data from one 1997 study are used to claim that mortality rates are lower among HIV positives treated with protease inhibitors.[77] This particular trial was prematurely terminated before statistically significant results could be obtained, and no placebo control comparing unmedicated HIV positives was used, no recurrent AIDS-defining illnesses that appeared among participants were recorded (except recurrent pneumonia), and the results mentioned in the final report are for only a small fraction of the patients enrolled in the study.[78] Current pharmaceutical ads use this study to declare that their new drugs are "proven to help people with HIV live longer, healthier lives" while simultaneously admitting that "because the study ended early, there was insufficient data to determine [the drug's] statistical impact on survival."[79]

While there is no evidence that cocktail therapies produce clinical health benefits, well-documented side effects include headache, fever, nausea, vomiting, diarrhea, oral lesions, abdominal pain, severe fatigue, sexual dysfunction, general ill feeling, skin rashes, a hypersensitivity reaction that can result in sudden death, nervous system damage, enlarged liver, liver failure, kidney stones, kidney sludge, physical deformities including hunchbacks, sunken cheeks, and "stick-like limbs," diabetes, heart disease, "unmasking" of various opportunistic infections including CMV retinitis (a viral infection which can lead to blindness), and spontaneous bleeding in hemophiliacs.[80]

Media reports attributing declines in AIDS to protease inhibitor cocktails often neglect to mention the high rate of drug failure or the considerable number of HIV positives who either quit the new combinations because of intolerable side effects or have never taken them at all. Recent studies place drug failure rates at 50% while others note that as many as 40% of participants drop out of protease inhibitor drug trials due to adverse effects, and as AIDS expert Dr. James Curran laments, "fewer than 10% of US AIDS patients have access to and are on the new wonder drugs."[81] For more information on the chemotherapy/protease inhibitor drug combinations known as HAART, please see *A Sobering Report on AIDS Cocktails* and *What's Up with Viral Load?* on pages 32 and 36.

9 Does HIV Take Years to Cause AIDS?

For more than a decade, scientists throughout the world agreed that HIV had a latency period, a time during which it remained inactive before becoming active and causing immune destruction. The notion of a latency period was used to explain why HIV did not behave like all other infectious, disease-causing microbes that cause illness soon after infection, and why significant quantities of active HIV could not be found in people who test HIV positive.

At first, HIV's latency period was thought to be a few months long.[82] It was then revised to one year, then two, then three and five years.[83] As greater numbers of people who tested HIV positive did not develop AIDS as predicted, the latency period was extended to ten or fifteen years, and more recently, even to entire lifetimes.[84]

Just when HIV's growing latency period became the focus of mounting scrutiny, it was replaced with the concept of constantly active HIV that replicates and destroys cells at spectacular rates, a hypothesis known as "viral load." The media, government health agencies, AIDS organizations, and most AIDS doctors have uncritically accepted the viral load concept as fact. Proponents of viral load assert that HIV is rampant and destructive from the very moment of infection, and that the immune system of a person who tests positive is engaged in a perpetual struggle to keep the virus under control. They claim that HIV, after five, ten or fifteen years, eventually wins the battle by wearing out the immune system.

Viral load relies entirely on conclusions drawn from **polymerase chain reaction (PCR)** tests, and is based on the erroneous notion that the fragments of genetic material PCR finds correspond to counts of actual virus. In fact, PCR is unable to detect actual virus; it only amplifies genetic material associated with HIV (RNA or DNA) and the "load" produced by the test is a mathematical calculation, not a count of infectious virus. When standard methods of virus counting are applied, a viral load of 100,000 has been shown to correspond to less than ten infectious units of HIV, an amount that is far too small to induce illness.[85]

Contrary to popular belief, PCR cannot determine what portion, if any, of the genetic material it detects represents infectious virus. In fact more than 99% of what PCR measures is noninfectious.[86] Dr. Kary Mullis, who won the 1993 Nobel Prize for inventing PCR is a member of The Group for the Scientific Reappraisal of the HIV/AIDS Hypothesis and refutes those who claim that HIV is the causative agent of AIDS.[87]

Viral loads have been measured in people who are HIV negative and in AIDS patients who test HIV antibody positive but have no HIV.[88] Low levels of viral load have not been correlated with good health, with absence of illness or high T cell counts while high viral loads do not correspond with low T cells or sickness.[89] For more information, please see *What's Up with Viral Load?* on page 36.

Polymerase chain reaction (PCR): A technique used to detect the presence of minute quantities of genetic material in the blood through replication of DNA or RNA.

10 Do Pregnant Women Who Test HIV Positive Give Their Babies AIDS?

At least 75% of babies born to HIV positive mothers will test HIV negative without medical intervention.[90] Studies have shown that for properly nourished HIV positive expectant mothers receiving regular prenatal care, over 90% of their children test negative with no drug therapy.[91] Mainstream medical experts acknowledge that children need up to 18 months to develop their own immune response and discard the antibodies passed on to them from their mothers, and note that HIV testing before 18 months of age does not yield conclusive results.[92] Despite this widely accepted fact, several states require mandatory HIV antibody testing for newborns in public hospitals.[93]

As explained previously, HIV antibody tests do not indicate the presence of actual virus and are unable to determine if the antibodies it detects are even HIV antibodies. Newer "viral load" tests do not detect actual virus and are not approved for diagnostic use. Even when administered after 18 months of age, neither test can determine if a child is actually infected with HIV. Despite these facts, the tests are routinely used to diagnose HIV infection in newborns and children. The results of these inaccurate and improperly applied tests are the basis for all claims regarding transmission rates of HIV from mother to child, and for declaring that a baby "has HIV."

Expectant mothers who test HIV positive are commonly advised to abort or to take AZT, a highly toxic chemical compound originally created for use as a cancer treatment. AZT works by blocking the formation of DNA—a process essential to sustaining life—and destroying all growing cells, particularly new cells produced in the bone marrow where the immune system is generated. AZT is a known **carcinogen**, **mutagen**, and **teratogen**, and until recently it was **contraindicated** for use during pregnancy.[94]

AZT was approved for expectant mothers based on the conclusions of a single trial, ACTG076, a trial sponsored by AZT's manufacturer. According to this study, transmission rates of HIV were 25.5% for infants of untreated mothers and 8.3% for children born to the AZT-treated women.

Carcinogen: Any agent capable of causing cancer such as asbestos fibers and high-energy radiation. Chemicals form the largest group of carcinogens.

Mutagen: Any physical or chemical agent that, when applied to a group of living cells, increases the rate of mutation in those cells. Mutation is a change in the genetic material within a cell which can give rise to cancer or a hereditary disease.

Teratogen: An agent that causes physical abnormalities in a developing embryo or fetus. The drug thalidomide is an example of a teratogen. Drug regulating agencies usually refuse to license drugs for use during pregnancy if they have been found to be teratogenic for any species.

Contraindicated: A line of medical treatment, such as drug therapy or surgery, that is inadvisable or unwise due to any factor in a patient's condition.

The results of ACTG076 have proved impossible to duplicate in further studies on pregnant women treated with AZT. In fact, other reports have shown that expectant mothers using prenatal multivitamins experienced lower rates of transmission than the lowest rate of those treated with AZT. One study determined that use of vitamin A correlates with a transmission rate of 7.2%.[95]

The effects of AZT on expectant mothers include muscle deterioration, severe anemia, nerve damage, liver damage, muscle wasting, lymphoma, acute nausea, diarrhea and dementia. The effects of AZT on developing infants include misshapen heads, extra fingers, triangular faces, albinism, misplaced ears, cavities in the chest, webbed fingers, anemia, spontaneous abortion, chromosomal damage, and can result in the need for therapeutic abortions of severely deformed fetuses.[96]

Routine HIV antibody testing for pregnant women raises particular concerns as pregnancy itself can cause positive HIV test results.[97] Although cross-reactions due to pregnancy are documented in the medical literature and acknowledged by test manufacturers, HIV antibody tests have become part of standard prenatal screening, and are even mandatory in some states.

A fundamental problem of routine screening using even the most accurate test is that low risk groups will have the highest rates of false positives. This occurs because the accuracy of a test deteriorates when administered to populations among which the microbe being tested for is rarely found. Since the incidence of HIV positivity among American women who describe themselves as risk-free is 0.01%, a consequence of routine HIV screening of all expectant women is widespread false positive results.[98] One study of premarital HIV screening reported that HIV antibody tests with an alleged specificity of 99.8% and sensitivity of 98.3% had an accuracy of less than 15% when administered to this low risk group.[99] And these figures are based on invalid and/or loose definitions of specificity, sensitivity, and accuracy that do not involve tests validated by identifying actual HIV infections.

Another troubling consequence of requiring HIV tests for pregnant women is the emerging issue of obligatory drug treatment. While CDC guidelines state that "discussion of treatment options should be non-coercive, and the final decision to accept or reject AZT for herself and her child is the right and responsibility of the woman," such discussions rarely include objective data on the toxic effects of AIDS drugs or any information that would support a decision to reject them.[100] Most health practitioners promote the notion that a positive test indicates infection with a lethal virus, and portray AIDS medication as particularly urgent and necessary for expectant women.

Although the CDC says that "a [mother's] decision not to accept treatment should not result in punitive action," suggested standards of care have been legally mandated in some instances and children have been taken from parents who choose not to accept treatment.[100] In one recent case, public health officials in Eugene, Oregon intervened when an HIV positive mother declined AZT therapy for her HIV negative infant son.[101] As a result of her decision, both parents were charged with neglect, and the state took legal custody of their healthy newborn boy who was given six weeks of AZT treatment.[102]

Another HIV positive mother in Bangor, Maine faced charges of "serious parental neglect" for declining to provide her son with AIDS drugs that had previously caused him harm.[103] Her four-year-old boy, HIV positive since birth, had become so anemic during 10 weeks of AIDS treatment as to require blood transfusions, and experienced a host of adverse effects that left him unable to walk and in almost continual pain.[104] His mother discontinued treatment after noting that his health returned when she stopped giving him the drugs. After a District Court found in her favor, an appeal was brought before the State Supreme Court challenging the decision. In this case, the mother was granted the right to keep her son off AIDS medications and in her custody.[105]

As this book went to press, authorities in Montreal, Canada seized the children of a woman who has been HIV positive, healthy and unmedicated for 13 years after she declined HIV treatment for her two boys. The Quebec Superior Court agreed to delay administration of drugs to her sons, ages three and seven, pending the determination of a custody hearing. The mother told the court that HIV treatments are experimental and highly toxic, and that her family has been healthy without using drugs.[106]

Whose Benefits Outweigh the Risks?

Documented effects of AZT, also known as Zidovudine, Retrovir-Zidovudine, and ZDV. AZT is also one of the two active ingredients in Combivir.

"HIV-1 infected children with mothers who were treated with zidovudine had a 'higher probability of developing severe disease' compared with untreated children. These children also had a higher probability of severe immune suppression and lower survival."

Reuters Health, June 2, 1999 on a report in the May 28, 1999 issue of *AIDS* 13:927-933

"Concerns are being fueled by a study from a team at the National Cancer Institute near Washington, DC. In the journal *AIDS* (Vol 13 p 919), the researchers report that AZT is incorporated into the DNA of white blood cells in people treated with the drug—including pregnant women and their babies. This is because AZT mimics thymidine, one of the four nucleosides that make up the genetic code. Olivero and her colleagues warn that the changes may increase the chance of developing cancer."

Michael Day, *New Scientist*, June 26, 1999

"In reviewing the frequency of birth defects in this population [of HIV positive women taking AZT during pregnancy] we noted eight birth defects (10%) out of 80 live births."

Kumar et al, Zidovudine Use in Pregnancy: A Report on 104 Cases and the Occurrence of Birth Defects, *Journal of AIDS*, Vol. 4, 1994

"Concerns stem from a study led by Stéphane Blanche of the Necker Hospital in Paris. He has examined the cases of around a thousand pregnant women with HIV and found that eight gave birth to babies who, though HIV-negative, suffered from a neurodegenerative condition that kills its victims in infancy. The condition highlighted by Blanche is thought to be caused by abnormalities in mitochondria, the energy 'factories' within our cells. The babies' mothers had all taken a combination of the drugs AZT and 3TC from week 32 of their pregnancy. This condition is an extraordinarily rare mitochondrial disorder that you might expect to see in only 1 in 10,000 or 1 in 100,000 births."

Michael Day, *New Scientist*, June 26, 1999

"At present, data regarding the effects of ZDV use on vertical [mother to child] transmission rates are inconclusive and incomplete. In addition, the long-term effects of ZDV use during pregnancy and after birth on the woman and any resulting child are yet to be discovered. The possibility has not yet been ruled out that this 'risk-reducing' measure may not be effective and may prove detrimental to the health of both mother and child."

Bennett, Mandatory Testing of Pregnant Women and Newborns: A Necessary Evil? *AIDS/STD Health Promotion Exchange*, 1998

"A total of 172 participants died [169 while taking AZT, 3 while on placebo]...The results of Concorde do not encourage the early use of zidovudine in symptom-free HIV-infected adults...Representatives of the Wellcome Foundation who were also members of the Coordinating Committee have declined to endorse this report."

Concorde Coordinating Committee, Concorde: MRC/ANRS Randomised Double-blind Controlled Trial of Immediate and Deferred Zidovudine in Symptom-free HIV Infection, *The Lancet*, Vol 343, April 9, 1994

"Following combination antiretroviral therapy administered during pregnancy, most HIV positive mothers and their children developed one or more adverse events, according to the results of an observational study.

"Dr. Lorenzi's group evaluated 37 pregnant women with HIV infection and the 30 infants who had been born at the time of the study. All of the women received two reverse transcriptase inhibitors, and 16 women were also given a protease inhibitor. Among the infants, the most common adverse event was prematurity (10 infants), followed by profound anemia (8 infants). The investigators also noted two cases of cutaneous angioma, two cases of cryptorchidism, and one case of transient hepatitis. Two infants whose mothers were on triple therapy with a protease inhibitor developed non-life-threatening intracerebral hemorrhage. One infant, also exposed to triple therapy, developed extrahepatic biliary atresia."

Reuters, January 1, 1999

" New York researchers report a case of severe anemia in a newborn infant that was probably caused by treatment of the HIV positive mother with the antiretroviral combination of zidovudine, lamivudine and zalcitabine. The male infant, who was pale and developed respiratory distress soon after birth, '...was diagnosed with high output congestive heart failure secondary to profound anemia.'

" Dr. Wendy J. Watson of the University of Rochester Medical Center and colleagues ruled out infection, nutritional deficiencies, congenital leukemia and congenital red blood cell aplasia in the child. 'The cause of the life-threatening anemia in our infant is presumed to be utero bone marrow suppression by one or more of the antiretroviral agents administered to the mother,' they report in the May issue of *The Pediatric Infectious Disease Journal*."

Reuters, June 8, 1998

" ...the estimated probability of developing [Non-Hodgkin's] lymphoma [in patients taking AZT alone, or in combination] by 30 months of therapy was 28.6%...and by 36 months, 46.4%."

Pluda et al, Development of Non-Hodgkin's Lymphoma in a Cohort of Patients with Severe Human Immunodeficiency Virus (HIV) Infection on Long-Term Antiretroviral Therapy, *Annals of Internal Medicine*, 1990; 113(4): 276-282

" The long-term consequences of in-utero and infant exposure to zidovudine are unknown. The long-term effects of early or short-term use of zidovudine in pregnant women are also unknown."

Retrovir, Canadian Pharmaceutical Association Compendium of Pharmaceuticals, 1997; 1357-1361

" A long-term federal government study of AZT begun in August 1991 involving 839 children at 62 hospitals was halted. An independent committee monitoring the trial recommended it be halted because 'the children receiving AZT had more rapid rates of disease progression, AIDS-related infections, impaired neurological development and death.'"

The New York Times, February 14, 1995

" Proven Power For HIV: Because of her baby, because she vows to be there for her family, because her kids remind her to take her combination of anti-HIV medicines everyday...There are no adequate and well-controlled studies of Combivir [lamivudine/zidovudine tablets] in pregnant women. Combivir should be used in pregnancy only if the potential benefits outweigh the risks."

Glaxo-Wellcome ad for Combivir, April 1999

AZT's manufacturer Glaxo-Wellcome reported $2.35 billion in annual sales of AZT and their other antiviral drugs for 1997.[107]

AZT: A Drug in Search of a Disease

AZT is not a new drug. It was not created for the treatment of AIDS and is not an antiviral. AZT is a chemical compound that was developed—and abandoned—over 30 years ago as a potential chemotherapy treatment for cancer.[108] Prior to the first AIDS drug trials in 1986, AZT had never been administered to human beings.

Chemotherapy works by killing all growing cells in the body. Many cancer patients do not survive chemotherapy due to its destructive effects on the immune system and intestines. Because of the damage it causes, chemotherapy is never used as a prevention for cancer, and is only administered for very limited amounts of time.

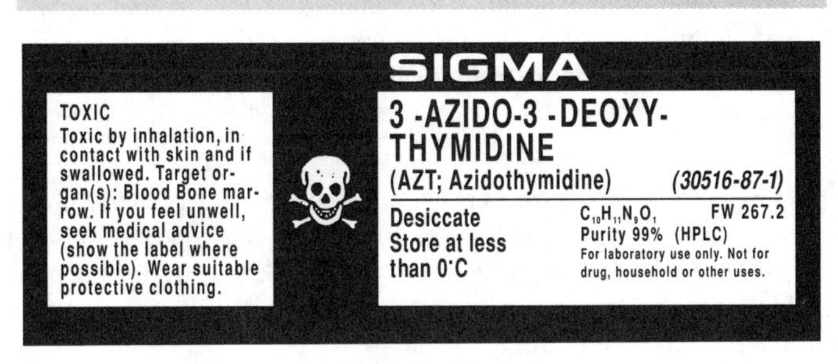

Copy of an AZT Label

This label has appeared on bottles containing as little as 25 milligrams, a small fraction (1/20 to 1/60) of a patient's daily prescribed dose of 500 to 1,500 mg.[109]

Since cancer is a condition of persistently growing cells, AZT was designed to prevent the formation of new cells by blocking development of DNA chains. In 1964, experiments with AZT on mice with cancer showed that AZT was so effective in destroying healthy growing cells that the mice died of extreme toxicity.[110] As a result, AZT was shelved and no patent was ever filed. Twenty years later, the pharmaceutical company Burroughs Wellcome (now Glaxo-Wellcome) began a campaign to remarket AZT as an anti-HIV drug based on the idea that AZT would block the formation of HIV DNA chains. Glaxo-Wellcome won FDA approval for AZT as an AIDS treatment after one highly flawed study of only four months duration.[111]

Approval of this extremely toxic chemotherapy for use by AIDS patients was based on information that suggested AZT raised levels of T cells and therefore delayed the onset of AIDS indicator diseases. The rise noted in T cells was interpreted as evidence that AZT eradicated HIV in T cells, a concept for which there is no scientific proof. Although the study was halted before any long-term effects of AZT were known, proponents established that standard treatment with AZT should be continuous and lifelong.

A multitude of independent studies conducted before and after FDA approval, including the Concorde study—the largest (1,749 subjects) and longest (three years in duration) study on AZT—determined that AZT increases T cell counts only moderately and briefly without improving health and that it does not delay onset of AIDS indicator diseases.[112]

The brief rise in T cells noted when AZT use is initiated is due to the toxic nature of the drug and to the blood system's response to the destruction of bone marrow.[113] As AZT destroys bone marrow, the blood system attempts to correct this depletion by overproducing T cells, often creating more new T cells than the number found in a patient's blood prior to beginning treatment. But as the source of these new T cells—the bone marrow—is killed off by AZT, the level of T cells drops lower, ultimately causing complete destruction of the immune system. Individual tolerance to, and absorption of AZT determine length of survival on this toxic compound.

Following recommendations for "early intervention," one-third to one-half of HIV positives who develop AIDS do so only after taking AZT. Independent studies have shown that AZT actually accelerates clinical decline and decreases quality of life, at times even causing death before any AIDS-defining illnesses appear—an occurrence officially described as "death without any preceding AIDS-defining event."[114]

The concept of "HIV mutation" has become a popular explanation for the fall in T cells observed in patients treated with AZT. Promoters of the mutation hypothesis assert that the positive effects of AZT are diminished by mutant strains of HIV that become resistant to the drug. There is, however, no scientific evidence to substantiate their claim.

AIDS by Prescription?[115]

The following conditions are caused by nucleoside analog drugs (AZT, ddI, ddC, D4T and 3TC). Conditions followed by a bullet (•) are official AIDS-defining illnesses:

- Anemia (requiring transfusions)
- Birth defects
- Diarrhea •
- Dementia •
- Fertility impairment
- **Granulocytopenia**
- Hair loss
- Headaches
- Liver damage
- Loss of appetite
- Lymphoma (cancer) •
- Muscle wasting •
- Nausea
- Neuropathy
- Pancreatitis
- **Pancytopenia**
- Seizures
- Skin discolorations
- Spontaneous abortion
- T cell depletion •

Granulocytopenia: Loss or reduction of the number of granulocytes, a group of white blood cells that fight infection. These white blood cells contain a variety of enzymes used to destroy infectious agents.

Pancytopenia: Generalized loss or reduction of white blood cells.

In addition to destroying T cells, **B cells** and the red blood cells that carry oxygen throughout the body, AZT and other **nucleoside analog** drugs destroy the kidneys, liver, intestines, muscle tissue, and the central nervous system. Nucleoside analog drugs also interfere with the activities of mitochondria, the subcellular particles that are the energy factories of every living cell in the body. Mitochondria contain their own DNA which makes them vulnerable to the effects of nucleoside analogs.

Epivir (3TC), Zerit (D4T), Hivid (ddC) and Videx (ddI) are all nucleoside analog drugs prescribed to HIV positives as "antivirals." All are modeled after AZT, and all work in the same manner.

B cells: One of two principle types of lymphocytes (white blood cells). B cells are transformed into plasma cells that secrete immunoglobulins or antibodies that destroy invading microorganisms. The protective effect of immunoglobulins is called humoral immunity.

Nucleoside analog: A synthetic compound similar to one of the components of DNA or RNA. Nucleoside analogs such as AZT act as artificial caps to DNA chains which prevent real DNA units from being added. For this reason these drugs are often referred to as DNA chain terminators.

A Sobering Report on Protease Inhibitors and "Combo Cocktails"

Protease inhibitors are a new class of AIDS drugs used in conjunction with older chemotherapy compounds such as AZT and ddI. The mixture of these treatments is called a "combination cocktail" or "highly active antiretroviral therapy" (HAART). The formula is usually two parts nucleoside analog to one part protease inhibitor. According to popular belief, this mix brings new power to the old chemotherapies, and achieves what press reports and AIDS groups characterize as unprecedented and amazing results.

Approved after the fastest and most lenient review process in FDA history and immediately hailed as miraculous by mainstream media, the clinical benefits of protease inhibitor drugs remain unproved. More than four years after being released for use, there are still no reports in scientific journals that provide evidence of health improvement in patients taking these powerful drugs.

Claims of victory for protease inhibitors are based entirely on changes in **surrogate markers**, laboratory measurements of unsubstantiated accuracy and value in assessing actual health. In the only published report alleging higher survival rates for patients treated with protease inhibitors, the study used no unmedicated placebo controls, did not allow reporting of any recurrent AIDS-defining events except pneumonia, included no patient data, cited outcomes for less than 10% of overall participants, and was prematurely terminated after an average follow-up of 38 weeks when emerging mortality statistics favored the protease inhibitor treated patients.[115] The survival outcomes between the two groups—1.4% mortality among those on the new drugs, 3.1% for the old drugs—have no statistical significance, a fact that forces the drug advertisements to admit "because the study was ended early, there was insufficient data to determine the statistical impact of Crixivan on survival."[117]

One National Institutes of Health study of protease inhibitors, ACTG 315, is portrayed as a success even though its conclusions are drawn from a trial of only 12 weeks.[118] Dr. Michael Lederman, protocol chairman and author of ACTG 315 acknowledged that the study was never designed to consider a patient's health. Instead, results were determined by changes in the surrogate marker of "viral load," a test that does not diagnose illness, quantify active virus or measure health.

The absence of data on long-term effects of protease inhibitors has not prevented orthodox AIDS organizations who promote or provide the drugs from becoming uncritical advocates. Following the lead of the media, their focus has been on securing widespread access to the treatments rather than on examining evidence to insure they are safe and effective. AIDS doctors have also overlooked the

Surrogate marker: A laboratory test result that takes the place of or substitutes for a clinical indication or diagnosis.

remarkable lack of documentation in favor of the options for treatment offered by protease inhibitors. And while boldface headlines continue to assign lifesaving properties to these drugs, the tiny type in pharmaceutical ads, the ever-growing list of side effects, and the increasing number of unsuccessful experiences—ranging from physical deformities to sudden death—tell an entirely different story.

Protease inhibitors are assumed to work by disrupting an enzymatic link in the reproduction of HIV. Enzymes are proteins that join together or cut apart other molecules. Like all retroviruses, HIV has three enzymes: reverse transcriptase, integrase, and protease which cut proteins apart, an essential step in the reproductive process of a retrovirus. Protease inhibitors block proteases by acting as dysfunctional molecules that take the place of functional ones and inhibit the cutting apart of proteins. All retroviral enzymes are similar to various human enzymes and there are numerous human proteases, including ones required for digestion of food.

Protease inhibitors are like nucleoside analog drugs such as AZT in that they produce dysfunctional substitutes that interrupt or prevent normal processes of enzymes. While manufacturers of protease inhibitors claim that the drugs specifically target HIV protease, the growing list of side effects contradicts their assertions. Nucleoside analogs such as AZT, once promoted as specifically targeting HIV, have been shown to block the construction of vital human DNA as effectively as they block the formation of HIV DNA. It is now known that AZT, ddI and other nucleoside analogs block the DNA inside mitochondria, the subcellar particles that produce the energy required for the life of all cells.

The necessity for lifelong therapy with protease inhibitor cocktails is described as absolute, although drug manufacturers clearly state that "the long-term effects of protease inhibitors are unknown." The need for rigorous compliance with combo therapy is a popular subject of news reports and AIDS organization seminars. Patients are required to pop as many as 30 pills a day on a 24 hour schedule—some taken with food, others on an empty stomach, many that cannot be taken together—and warned that without strict adherence to the dosages and times, their virus will mutate into new, drug resistant strains.

According to Dr. David Rasnick, a protease expert working outside the AIDS system, the theory of resistant HIV protease is completely unfounded. Rasnick, a pioneer in the development of protease inhibitors points out, "no one has ever published data on a resistant HIV protease found in any patient. The only inhibitor-resistant HIV proteases ever examined have been produced in the lab using genetic engineering."[119]

Nevertheless, warnings about drug-resistant HIV proteases are emphasized in media reports that also speculate about new epidemics that will arise when unstoppable forms of HIV are introduced into the population. As announced by AIDS researcher Dr. Bruce Walker on a recent segment of ABC News' *Nightline*, "That's going to be the next epidemic that we're dealing with, the transmission of drug resistant HIV viruses."[120] Such reports reinforce the notion that no matter how unbearable the side effects, a patient who quits the drugs becomes a public health menace. This science-fiction scenario has even inspired some health officials and legislators to consider mandatory treatment laws for HIV positives.[121]

Perhaps the greatest achievement of protease inhibitors is the new life they have given to AIDS advertising campaigns. An epidemic of posters, billboards, and full-page magazine ads urge HIV positives to "be smart about HIV" by "hitting early and hard" with medicines "proven to help people live longer, healthier lives."[122] However, many staunch supporters of AIDS pharmaceuticals are less certain. Top AIDS scientist Dr. Anthony Fauci expressed serious reservations about the use of protease inhibitors by "otherwise healthy people" in a recent article in the *Journal of the American Medical Association*, "We do not know whether early intervention in asymptomatic individuals will result in a long-term clinical benefit or whether the cumulative toxicity over years of drug administration will outweigh the potential benefits."[123] Even Dr. Robert Gallo has warned that "these drugs are toxic...the longer you take the drugs, the greater the toxicity."[124] Dr. Jay Levy, another mainstream AIDS specialist, maintains that "these drugs can be toxic and can be directly detrimental to a natural immune response to HIV."[125]

A careful examination of the small print in protease inhibitor ads puts the promises made by smiling models into perspective: "Since Crixivan has been marketed, other side effects have been reported including rapid breakdown of red blood cells, kidney stones and kidney failure. In some patients with hemophilia, increased bleeding has been associated with protease inhibitor use."[126] Pre-marketing side effects like diarrhea, nausea, fungal infections, bloody urine, weakness, headaches and liver inflammation were all but ignored by AIDS activists who pressured the FDA for fast-track approval.[127] The list of post-marketing side effects continues to grow and contradicts earlier reports on the cocktails that proclaimed, "It's unbelievable. There's no toxicity. It's a home run!"[128]

Documented adverse reactions presently include CMV retinitis (a viral infection that often results in blindness), diabetes, liver failure, physical deformities, renal failure, kidney sludge, skin rashes, severe exhaustion, loss of appetite, **pancreatitis**, diarrhea, nausea and vomiting, muscle and joint pain, **neuropathy**, sexual dysfunction, fever, chills, dizziness, abdominal pain, depression, sleep disorders, and sudden death.[129]

Other than anecdotal tales of miraculous recoveries trumpeted in the press, the lower levels of "viral load" found in some patients taking protease cocktails seem to be the only and highly questionable result of these treatments. But even "undetectable" viral loads are not an unprecedented occurrence in HIV treatment—AZT has lowered those levels for many years without resolving AIDS. A *POZ* magazine article recalls that "in the European Delta study, fully 40% of participants became 'undetectable' [for viral load] on AZT/ddI; another 5% did so on AZT alone. We have been reducing viral load to undetectable levels for a decade. But if becoming 'undetectable' on nucleoside combos hasn't prevented progression to disease and death, why is 'undetectable' on protease combinations impervious to failure—except for the fact that we haven't followed patients long enough to see it?"[130]

Although the media credits "AIDS cocktails" with recent decreases in AIDS cases and deaths, CDC surveillance reports clearly show that AIDS cases and mortalities began declining before the cocktails were approved for use.[131]

Pancreatitis: Inflammation of the pancreas; chronic pancreatitis often causes diabetes.

Neuropathy: Any disease or disorder of the nervous system.

Some experts attribute the drops in AIDS deaths to the fact that over half of all AIDS cases reported since 1993 are among people who test HIV positive but have no illness or symptoms.[132] The same reports show that AIDS cases had leveled off in 1991 and increased only once since, in the first quarter of 1993 when more conditions and illness were added to the definition of AIDS.

For some, the chorus of enthusiastic press reports about protease inhibitors recalls the release of AZT twelve years ago. "Once again, all we have are researchers talking to reporters about incomplete studies that haven't been scrutinized by the scientific review process," remarks Dr. Rasnick. "And the researchers involved are funded by the companies that make the drugs in question. There is no justification for the claims coming from these sources, particularly when we've seen it all before."[133]

Declarations of success and improved survivability for AZT were based on abbreviated trials of less than six months duration that were sponsored by the drug's manufacturer who selected for publication only those trials with seemingly favorable outcomes. Success was measured by the surrogate marker of that day, increased T cell counts, which have proved to be a temporary phenomenon at best and of questionable clinical value. As with AZT, the elation unleashed over protease inhibitors is based on unpublished manufacturers' studies so brief they are usually measured in weeks rather than months, and on the surrogate marker of reduced "viral load," a measurement that has not been correlated with actual health benefits. While the media persists with stories of the miraculous achievements of protease inhibitors making believers out of the concerned public and desperate AIDS patients, only time and independent research will reveal the truth about the latest "great hope" in the war on AIDS.

Reasons to Wonder About the Wonder Drugs[134]

- There are no long-term studies that demonstrate health benefits or increased life expectancy for patients taking the drug combinations known as HAART.
- Studies show that HAART actually shuts down numerous functions of the immune system considered essential for survival including the activity of many cytokines, proteins that trigger vital immune responses.
- 30% of patients taking HAART suffer from lipodystrophy, a fat distribution and metabolic disorder that can lead to heart attacks and strokes, and cause fat lumps known as "buffalo humps" and other physical deformities.
- The decreased levels of viral load that occur in some patients taking HAART do not correlate with wellness, increased T cells or improved rates of survival.

What's Up with Viral Load?

One glaring problem with the HIV/AIDS hypothesis is that researchers have been unable to find enough HIV (actual virus) in people who test positive to explain compromised health. Even among patients suffering from the most severe AIDS-defining illnesses, HIV is never detected in quantities that could cause depletion of immune cells.[135]

In order to cause harm, a virus needs to infect at least one-third of all target cells, which in the case of AIDS are the T cells of the immune system, and kill these cells faster than they can be replaced. For example, with hepatitis or a common cold or flu, the responsible virus is readily found in quantities measuring millions or billions per milliliter (mL) of blood, and nothing can stop the virus from infecting all susceptible cells in the body except antiviral immunity. With AIDS, an average of only ten HIVs are found per mL of blood, and the normal sign of antiviral immunity, antibodies, are said to indicate illness.[136]

Another inconsistency with the idea that HIV causes AIDS is that HIV is non-cytotoxic. This means that when HIV replicates, it does not kill the host cell. Other viruses that cause disease are cytotoxic; they destroy the cell they infect when they reproduce, and rapidly claim 30% to 60% of target cells. Since the acceptance of HIV as the cause of AIDS in 1984, AIDS researchers have proposed a multitude of hypotheses about HIV's ability to provoke cell destruction through elaborate and as yet unproven indirect mechanisms while searching in vain for ways to explain how a non-cytotoxic virus can eliminate T cells and cause AIDS.

For almost a decade, the latency notion was used to justify some of the paradoxical qualities attributed to HIV. Experts claimed that HIV was a slow virus that remained inactive or latent for a period of time before becoming active and destroying immune cells. This idea gained universal acceptance despite the fact that significant quantities of HIV were not found when HIV should have been at its most active—when AIDS patients are acutely ill.[137]

The loose ends of the HIV hypothesis were finally thought to have been tied in 1995 with two papers by a team of AIDS researchers led by Dr. David Ho of the Aaron Diamond Research Center and Dr. George Shaw of the University of Alabama. Ho and Shaw offered what they characterized as indisputable evidence that HIV is active from the moment of infection, and present in quantities sufficient to cause massive T cell destruction.[138] They claimed to find an average of over 100,000 HIVs per mL of blood in AIDS patients by using a virus counting method based on the new technology of polymerase chain reaction (PCR).

Their papers asserted that HIV has always been present and active in enormous quantities, but that its presence and activity could not be measured by standard means, and that scientists were looking for the wrong thing to measure. Until 1995, the method for finding and quantifying a virus was by isolation of the virus. This simple, direct method has been successfully applied to every virus except HIV. Instead, proponents of viral load assert that scientists must look for fragments of genetic materials rather than isolating the virus.

PCR is an innovative technique that enables scientists to take a sample of blood containing an otherwise undetectable number of DNA or RNA molecules and produce detectable quantities of fragments from these few original molecules. *Forbes* magazine described PCR as "biotechnology's version of the Xerox machine." Dr. Kary Mullis, who won a Nobel Prize for this revolutionary creation, explains that "PCR makes it possible to identify a needle in a haystack by turning the needle into a haystack."[139] While PCR has provided many realms of science and industry with an effective new tool, its application to AIDS research has been far more misleading than useful.

Ho and other researchers employed PCR to find, not HIV, but fragments of RNA, the genetic material in the viral core. Using the logic that each HIV virus particle contains two HIV RNAs, they assumed that every two RNA pieces indicated by PCR must correspond to one HIV viral particle, and they called the sum of what is copied, multiplied, counted, and divided, "viral load."

Viral load has been celebrated in the press as an astounding breakthrough in AIDS research, and has won Dr. David Ho numerous awards including *Time* magazine's 1996 Man of the Year. Viral load is also the measure by which new AIDS drugs are deemed effective. Protease inhibitors were approved for use based solely on their alleged ability to reduce "viral load." The media, AIDS organizations and most AIDS doctors have uncritically accepted the viral load hypothesis as fact.

According to the viral load hypothesis, billions of HIV are busy infecting CD4 T cells every day from the moment a person is exposed, and killer immune cells (CD8 T cells) continuously destroy billions of CD4 cells that host active HIV infection, while new, uninfected CD4s quickly replace the billions destroyed by the killer cells.[140] Eventually, after one to 15 years of this microscopic battle, the virus wears out the immune system allowing AIDS-defining illnesses to develop. Proponents of viral load claim that the reason this incredible activity was never noticed before is that the CD4s replicate so quickly, few HIV infected T cells ever make it into the blood where they can be measured.[140]

However, the viral load hypothesis fails to answer two important and unsettling questions: If billions of HIV are present, why is PCR necessary to find them? And if PCR is the only way HIV can be detected, how is it possible for scientists to verify the results of PCR?

Another problem with viral load is that PCR detects and multiplies single genes, not virus, and most often only fragments of genes. When it detects two or three genetic fragments out of a possible dozen complete genes, this is not proof that all the genes or the complete **genome** are present, or that a complete HIV viral particle is present.[141] Further, a person can carry a whole retroviral genome in their cells for an entire lifetime without ever producing a single virus.

The FDA has not approved PCR viral load for HIV screening or for diagnostic purposes. The CDC acknowledges that the specificity and sensitivity of PCR are "unknown" and that "PCR is not recommended and is not licensed for routine diagnostic purposes."[142] The viral load test manufacturers' literature

Genome: A biochemical map or blueprint; the complete set of hereditary factors as contained in a single set of chromosomes.

warn "the test is not intended to be used as a screening test for HIV or as a diagnostic test to confirm the presence of HIV..."[143]

Although no research has specifically studied PCR tests on HIV negative subjects, the medical literature records many incidents of detectable levels of viral load found in persons who are HIV negative.[144]

A group of AIDS researchers from the Johns Hopkins School of Public Health recently lamented the inaccuracies of PCR viral load, describing the test as unreliable and expensive when several attempts to verify PCR produced conflicting results.[145] A recent paper by AIDS reappraiser Dr. David Rasnick published in the *Journal of Biological Chemistry* demonstrates that at least 99.8% of what viral load tests measure are noninfectious virus particles, and notes that PCR should be replaced by a test that measures actual HIV in blood plasma.[146]

Can You Count on Viral Load?

- Viral load tests detect and multiply only fragments of genes, not HIV.
- Test manufacturers warn that viral load cannot confirm the presence of HIV.
- The FDA has not approved viral load tests for diagnostic use.
- Viral loads are found in healthy people who test HIV negative.
- High viral loads do not correlate with low T cells or illness.
- Low viral loads do not correlate with high T cells or wellness.

Although PCR viral load tests are unable to distinguish infectious virus from bits of noninfectious genetic fragments, are incapable of measuring actual virus, and are not approved for diagnostic use, the tests are being used by AIDS doctors every day to diagnose infection with HIV and as a basis for prescribing long-term treatment with protease inhibitors, chemotherapy compounds like AZT, powerful antibiotics and other drugs. PCR is routinely used to diagnose HIV infection in newborns, and as justification to treat infants with AZT, Bactrim and other potent chemicals.

PCR measurements do not correlate with amounts of T cells, with clinical symptoms of AIDS, or with levels of co-culturable HIV.[147] In the only published study that compares viral load results with the detection of HIV by **co-culture**,

Co-culture: Detection of a virus in an artificial laboratory environment that contains replicating microorganisms or cells mixed with plasma or immune cells.

a process that can artificially induce production of virus even when the patient's blood contains no virus, 53% of HIV positive AIDS patients with detectable levels of viral load—many with loads topping 200,000 and 300,000—had zero co-culturable HIV.[147]

A number of mainstream AIDS experts refute Ho's portrait of wildly multiplying and abundant HIV. Their objections have been published in *Nature, Lancet* and other science journals. Some, like former government AIDS researcher Dr. Cecil Fox dismiss Ho's ideas as "unconfirmed mathematical speculation."[148] According to orthodox AIDS expert Dr. Michael Asher, "the numbers [of the viral load theory] just don't add up."[148] Another prominent AIDS specialist, Dr. Mario Roderer, considers the viral load model of HIV **pathogenesis** a dead issue since "several well-designed and informative studies provide the final nails in the coffin for...the two *Nature* papers," while noted AIDS researcher Dr. Jay Levy warns that "medicine suffers when one is misled by numbers that are not relevant to the clinical problem involved..."[149] Other critics have been more blunt, characterizing this new hypothesis of HIV as "a viral load of crap."[150]

Pathogenesis: The process by which a disease or disorder originates and develops. Pathogenesis applies particularly to the cellular and physiological events involved in these processes.

Where's the HIV?

In accepting Gallo's AIDS virus hypothesis, researchers and physicians took for granted that Gallo had isolated a unique retrovirus, HIV, and that the proteins he used to construct the HIV antibody tests came from pure isolates of the virus. Since the announcement of Gallo's discovery of HIV however, a number of scientists have raised serious questions about what have been accepted as HIV isolates.

According to their claims, HIV, unlike other viruses, has never been isolated as an independent stable particle.[151] These scientists assert that electron microscope pictures or micrographs of all HIV isolates originally produced by Gallo and by other AIDS researchers since show some objects that look like retroviruses along with a number of other microbial objects that clearly are not viruses, and that among these, the retrovirus-like objects called HIV are only observed in cell cultures that have been stimulated by certain chemicals.[152]

Isolation is the only direct and unambiguous evidence of a virus, and isolation of a virus from the uncultured **plasma** of a patient is the only proof that a person has an active viral infection.[153] Cultures are artificial laboratory environments that contain replicating microorganisms or cells.

Normally, true isolation can be achieved without difficulty as people with an active viral infection will have lots of viruses in their plasma. This is not the case with HIV. In fact, there is no evidence that anyone has ever found what is called HIV in fresh plasma. Instead, AIDS researchers are only able to find what they call HIV when plasma or immune cells (co-cultures) and stimulating chemicals are added to cultures. Since artificially stimulated cultures can induce viral DNA to produce viruses even when the patient's plasma contains no virus, finding virus under these circumstances does not constitute evidence that patient plasma contains virus. True virus isolation requires using fresh, uncultured plasma.

When virus can be isolated from the fresh plasma of 99% of people who test positive in validation studies, the test can be considered 99% accurate. When claims of co-culture isolation are used to evaluate positive HIV test results, the accuracy is 0 to 10% for patients with no AIDS symptoms, and about 40% for patients who have symptoms of AIDS-defining illness. [154]

The true accuracy of HIV antibody tests has never been established by determining what percentage of people who test positive on HIV antibody tests have actual HIV that can be isolated from their fresh, uncultured plasma. This, along with the fact that what is called HIV has been observed only in artificial laboratory growths stimulated by chemical agents, has led some scientists to conclude that HIV has never been isolated and that all HIV tests are invalid.

Readers interested in further information on the isolation of HIV are encouraged to examine articles available at *www.virusmyth.com.*

Plasma: The natural solution that remains when white blood cells are removed from the blood.

Are These Facts News to You?

Why are we not getting all the facts about HIV and AIDS? Why do media reports uncritically promote HIV testing and the notion that everyone is at risk for AIDS? Why do the AIDS organizations supported by our tax dollars and donations leave the information addressed in this book out of their education programs and advertising campaigns? Some answers to these questions may be found by examining our current AIDS funding and research systems which offer little incentive for critical review, forthright discussion and innovation, but which are the source of most AIDS news.

Total tax dollars spent on AIDS presently exceeds $50 billion. Annual AIDS funding increases every year and is one of the only areas of the federal budget that has faced no threat of cuts. The high priority given to AIDS is based on the notion that AIDS poses a widespread and ever-growing health threat to all Americans. Since the government institutions responsible for generating official AIDS reports are the recipients of these multi-billions in AIDS dollars, it is understandable that the information they disseminate would support, rather than challenge the idea that AIDS is a large and growing problem. Their official reports are the basis for most AIDS news—reports that are not analyzed or investigated before they are repeated by the media and AIDS groups.

Investigative media reports on AIDS are generally discouraged because of sensitivity to the many social and political issues that surround HIV and AIDS. AIDS awareness, AIDS drugs, safe sex, and HIV testing are among the myriad concepts about AIDS that have been integrated into popular culture. Widespread acceptance of these concepts makes challenges to current views on HIV and AIDS appear highly controversial or even too dangerous to report. As orthodox AIDS expert and Nobel Laureate Dr. David Baltimore has declared, "There is no question HIV is the cause of AIDS. Anyone who gets up publicly and says the opposite is encouraging people to risk their lives."[155]

The Los Angeles Times recently acknowledged the factors that can influence AIDS news in "Protest Averted," an article that recounts the decision by a local TV station to alter a broadcast that mentioned decreases in AIDS: "After being pressured by the Los Angeles Gay and Lesbian Community Services Center, KCBS-TV Channel 2 has revised a station editorial on AIDS, deleting the line that stated 'A new report by the CDC indicates that AIDS is down in all categories and is not an epidemic.'"[156]

Many AIDS activist organizations charge that critical examination of HIV and AIDS is equivalent to promoting unsafe sex and may cause HIV positives to stop or refuse necessary pharmaceutical treatment. One such group, the San Francisco based drug advocacy organization Project Inform, brought their concerns regarding AIDS critics before the National Academy of Sciences. Project Inform's founder, Martin Delaney, is a nationally recognized AIDS activist and a member of the National Institute of Allergy and Infectious Diseases (NIAID) Council on AIDS. The group's National Board of Governors includes

HIV codiscoverer Dr. Robert Gallo and award-winning AIDS researcher Dr. David Ho. In 1997, Delaney petitioned the Academy asking them to expel members who engage in public challenges to the HIV=AIDS paradigm.[157]

In his letter to the Academy, Delaney denounces scientists who make information that questions AIDS available to "young and poorly informed people struggling with HIV infection [whose] natural inclination toward denial gives them a seemingly legitimate way to ignore a positive HIV antibody test, to cast aside...safe sex, and to forgo the complex challenge of multi-drug combination therapy." He suggests that AIDS is an area of public health that should not be examined in public forums, reasoning that "just as the blanket of free speech doesn't sanction the person who yells 'fire' in a crowded theater, neither does academic freedom provide protection for irresponsible behavior by scientists," and draws a parallel to criminal behavior claiming that "it is difficult to distinguish [the] actions [of scientists who raise questions about AIDS] from those of a mass murderer."

Attached to Project Inform's appeal is a list of supporting endorsements. Among the individuals and organizations joining the campaign to curtail critical discussion of AIDS science are AIDS Project Los Angeles; the Center for AIDS Prevention Studies at the University of San Francisco AIDS Research Institute; FAIR (Foundation for AIDS and Immune Research); the Florida AIDS Action Council; the United Foundation for AIDS; the Multicultural AIDS Coalition Inc.; Being Alive; Test Positive Aware Network; Gregory Britt, CEO of AIDS Research Alliance; noted AIDS researcher Dr. Michael Gottlieb; Brenda Freiberg, Chair of Public Policy at AIDS Service Center in Pasadena, California; Mary Lucey, President of Women Alive; and Dr. Martin Markowitz of the renowned Aaron Diamond Research Center in New York.

Project Inform's stance against information that questions AIDS is not unusual. For example, LA Shanti Foundation, a Los Angeles support network for people diagnosed with life-threatening illness, recently took a position on what many regard as life-affirming information about AIDS: My request to be considered as a speaker for their Positive Living For Us seminar, "a weekend for those who have tested positive for HIV...in which experts provide information about treatments, nutrition, sexuality, peer support, public benefits, insurance, legal matters, and other relevant topics," was not only rejected, my letter of inquiry was forwarded to the FDA's California AIDS Fraud Task Force, and to the District Attorney's AIDS Fraud Unit by the PLUS program manager, Ric Parish.[158] When asked by *The Valley Advocate* newspaper for comments on the growing movement to rethink AIDS, Nancy MacNeill, program coordinator for the Los Angeles AIDS group Women Alive exclaimed, "We hate them. They're spreading dangerous information."[159] Greg Gonsalves, founder of the New York City AIDS drug advocacy organization Treatment Action Group declared that "*SPIN* magazine's AIDS column is a public health menace" for its inclusion of alternative perspectives on AIDS.[160] Imposing limits on what AIDS information may be brought before the public limits public awareness of different ideas about HIV and AIDS.

AIDS organizations that object to public questioning of AIDS science may take their lead from mainstream media venues where news that challenges common perceptions about AIDS is rare. Journalists who cover AIDS seldom engage in investigative reporting and many have built successful careers by reiterating official AIDS views. Uncritical AIDS reports are the ones that have earned awards and have afforded many writers celebrity status. Laurie Garrett of *Newsday*, for example, has received two Pulitzer Prizes for her coverage of AIDS and frequently appears on television alongside prominent AIDS researchers and government health officials. In a recent issue of *Esquire* magazine, Garrett described the PCR test—a test not indicated or approved for the detection of HIV and unable to measure actual virus—as measuring HIV with "exquisite specificity."[161] Rather than rock the boat propelled by establishment AIDS views, high-level AIDS reporters generally dismiss or ignore challenges to the HIV=AIDS hypothesis.

Since the publications designed to reach HIV positives are funded almost entirely by AIDS drug manufacturers, it is not surprising that critical reporting on AIDS is absent from these venues. To cite just one example, AIDS pharmaceutical promotions filled 17 out of 31 pages allocated for advertisements in a current issue of *A&U: America's AIDS Magazine*. Of the remaining 14 pages, nine were purchased by viatical settlement groups offering cash in exchange for the life insurance policies of HIV positives.[162]

The research labs that produce the studies and reports that are turned into AIDS news all rely on some form of federal AIDS funding. Since the late 1980s, government support for AIDS research has been predicated on adherence to the HIV hypothesis. Institutions that depend on government dollars for support must assume that HIV is the cause of AIDS, and grants are not available to scientists or clinicians whose work may challenge the HIV hypothesis. For example, no funding has been provided for studies that compare the health of medicated and unmedicated HIV positives in matched control groups, for conducting viral load tests and T cell counts on HIV negatives matched to AIDS risk groups, or for verifying the accuracy of HIV antibody tests through isolation of actual virus in people with positive test results.

One well-known casualty of the AIDS funding system is Dr. Peter Duesberg of the University of California at Berkeley. Federal support for his laboratory was not renewed after his 1987 article in *Cancer Research* that questioned Gallo's HIV hypothesis and proposed an alternative AIDS hypothesis.[163] Before 1987, Duesberg received ongoing funding as a recipient of the NIH's prestigious Outstanding Investigator Award. He was also a Nobel candidate for his discovery of oncogenes, and is a member of the National Academy of Sciences. Since raising challenges to the HIV hypothesis, Duesberg has had 21 consecutive research grant applications rejected by the NIH and other federal and state funding sources.[164]

Pharmaceutical company grants are another important source of AIDS research money that make objective circumstances for drug studies almost impossible to achieve. Surprisingly, it is not considered a conflict of interest when AIDS researchers own stock in the companies whose products they test, or when they are hired to run the drug trials they publish in medical journals. In fact, it is common practice for drug companies to pay researchers to author favorable articles about their products.[165]

Many AIDS scientists previously employed by the US government have gone into private AIDS enterprise, a practice that further blurs the lines between news, public relations, and private interests. For example, the former director of the US Centers for Disease Control, Dr. Donald Francis, used his reputation in government AIDS work and his access to the media to raise $40 million in private investment capital for his AIDS vaccine company VaxGen.[166] In a recent CNN report on VaxGen, Francis promoted an AIDS vaccine as "the only way to stop a virus that is essentially 100 percent fatal."[167] In fact, most media stories that incite fear of AIDS and praise AIDS drugs derive from press releases or studies generated by AIDS drug developers. Since the pharmaceutical industry, like any other profit-oriented business, seeks to increase sales and profitability, expand its consumer base, and maintain a favorable public image, it is understandable that their press releases would promote continued success rather than provide critical or unfavorable information. However, their press releases are rarely questioned or scrutinized before being reported as news.

While America's institutions of higher learning are considered appropriate arenas for exploration of new ideas, open debate and discussion, this is often not the case when it comes to AIDS. To take just one recent example, members of the Graduate Students Council at Einstein College of Medicine in New York were discouraged from having their invited guest, Dr. Peter Duesberg, speak on campus. After being voted the student-selected speaker over orthodox AIDS researcher Dr. David Baltimore, and NIH Director Dr. Harold Varmus, Duesberg was informed that faculty members had pressured students into canceling the event. As student council chairman Robert Glover explained, "The general consensus is that many people would be offended by Duesberg's visit."[168]

As AIDS advocacy and service providers have grown from grassroots groups into multimillion dollar corporations, it has become harder for leaders to consider new ideas and approaches to resolving AIDS. For example, the success formula for the $45 million nonprofit AIDS Health Care Foundation of Los Angeles is providing AIDS drugs to people who test HIV positive.[169] Also, much of the money spent by AIDS groups comes from grants by pharmaceutical companies. To take just one example, the Washington, DC based National Association of People with AIDS receives funding from Merck, Glaxo-Wellcome, Roche, and Bristol-Myers Squibb.[170] Such situations provide little incentive for challenging popular ideas about HIV and AIDS.

There are an estimated 90,000 AIDS organizations in the US, about one for every six Americans ever given a diagnosis of AIDS.[171] Few, if any, of these groups evaluate the news they pass on to us in their education and awareness campaigns. Most repeat unexamined press releases from government agencies, the pharmaceutical industry and government-funded labs to the exclusion of all other information. And most will not participate in public discussion of the questions raised in this book.

Over 100 AIDS groups, AIDS specialists and researchers have declined my invitation to engage in a public dialogue on the validity of the HIV/AIDS hypothesis, the accuracy of HIV tests, and the safety and efficacy of AIDS treatment drugs. Their names are posted on the Alive & Well Alternatives website at *www.aliveandwell.org.*

Public Health, Public Relations, and AIDS

After nearly two decades of warnings about the impending heterosexual AIDS epidemic, none has materialized. In contrast to the dire predictions and despite widespread HIV testing, AIDS has remained almost exclusively confined to the original risk groups.[172] Even within risk groups, the numbers have never reached expected proportions and have been quietly diminishing for over five years. As AIDS in America has failed to live up to its terrifying reputation, our attention is directed to other parts of the world where harrowing estimates go unchecked and vastly exceed actual diagnoses.[173]

Information from the US Centers for Disease Control reveals that the disparity between official AIDS reports and actual AIDS data began in 1987. At that time, public health agencies elected to ignore their own findings in favor of promoting the notion that "everyone is at risk for AIDS."[174,175] Although epidemiology indicated this claim was not and would probably never be true, marketing research concluded that widespread support for AIDS would be impossible unless AIDS was considered a widespread health threat. Responding to Gallup Polls and PR studies, the CDC decided on a strategy that disregarded the facts in order to "mobilize support for public funding."[175] As CDC virologist Dr. Walter Dowdle admitted, "As long as this was seen as a gay disease, or even worse, a disease of drug abusers, this pushed the disease way down the ladder" of funding priorities.

The CDC's early decision to overestimate AIDS and magnify the risks launched one of the most successful advertising campaigns in history. In 1986, the majority of Americans did not feel at risk for AIDS; by 1988 more than two-thirds thought a full scale epidemic was likely, and by 1991, most believed that even married couples faced a substantial risk of contracting AIDS.[175] Federal tax dollars allocated to AIDS doubled the first year of the CDC ad campaign, and by the early 90s had topped $1 billion a year.

While concern and support for AIDS has multiplied and spread among millions of Americans, AIDS itself has not. This discrepancy has required a careful management of information and the need for constant advertisements, predictions and news reports that perpetuate ideas about AIDS that are out of sync with reality. Instead of revealing hard numbers and cold facts, most public health and AIDS organizations, along with the media, dispense reports that employ misleading percentages, alarming estimates, or cumulative totals for AIDS that disguise the realities of the epidemic.

The use of cumulative totals makes it possible to cite ever-growing numbers for AIDS even as AIDS is actually declining. Until 1997, despite steady decreases that began four years earlier, AIDS in America was almost universally described as an increasing problem, an image supported by the use of cumulative case numbers. For example, the total of new adult AIDS cases in the US in 1996 was 5,000 less than in 1995, but by adding the 1996 cases to the total number of cases reported since 1981, the decline of 5,000 was portrayed as an increase.[176]

Percentage calculations can turn drops into rises and are frequently used to make small numbers appear impressive. For example, in 1998 the number of new cases of AIDS among women decreased by more than 2,000, but at the same time, the percentage of total cases that women represent increased by 1%. This 1% difference in percentage is used to make the claim that AIDS is increasing among women.[176] The warning that heterosexuals are the fastest growing AIDS risk group is based on this same misleading use of percentages. In fact, cases of AIDS have been declining in all risk groups since 1993.[177]

Such statistical sleight of hand is not exclusive to the US media or American AIDS organizations. In Canada, a nation with an extremely low incidence of AIDS, government AIDS officials and the media play up the few cases there are and often perform their own magic with the numbers. For example, in 1995 new AIDS diagnoses among Canadian women totaled 175. This figure dropped to 165 in 1996, and then to 88 in 1997. News reports did not celebrate these decreases or the fact that in a country with some 15 million females, only 88 women were diagnosed with AIDS that year. Instead, the increased percentage of cases among women, from 8.8% of all AIDS cases in 1995 to 15.4% of AIDS cases in 1997, led Canada's Laboratory Centre for Disease Control (LCDC) to pronounce that women with AIDS made up "the highest proportion [of AIDS cases] observed since monitoring of the epidemic began."[178]

Estimates that can make anything seem possible are commonly used in AIDS news reports and advertising campaigns, and although the word "estimate" is crucial to qualifying claims, it is often omitted from ads and media reports. To take just one example, advertisements for the "Until There's A Cure" AIDS bracelet use blood-red capital letters to proclaim "16,000 people a day are introduced to HIV by testing positive."[179] It is necessary to contact the bracelet company in order to learn that the figure cited in the ad is an approximation based on global WHO estimates which are not even based on HIV test results.[180]

WHO estimates for AIDS in developing areas of the world such as Africa are the basis for many news reports. Although these estimates bear little resemblance to actual numbers of AIDS cases, the discrepancy might understandably be explained by the need to estimate a certain amount of AIDS cases in undiagnosed persons. However, the ratio of diagnosed cases to estimated cases inexplicably varies among African nations, ranging from nine estimated AIDS cases for every one case diagnosed, to as high as 69 for each single case.[181] For example, the WHO ratio for AIDS in Zimbabwe is 10/1, while the ratio of 48/1 is used next door in Mozambique, which changes to 33/1 across the border in neighboring South Africa.

Estimates are often combined with predictions, a mix that can produce particularly spectacular results. One recent example is a Reuters news release that announced "China has an estimated 400,000 people with HIV although confirmed cases [since the beginning of the epidemic] are only about 11,000." In this same report, "unidentified experts" went on to predict that these 11,000 cases could grow to "one million by the end of next year."[182]

Can Popular Consensus Be Wrong?

Throughout history, the medical and scientific communities have been in near unanimous agreement on causes and treatments for diseases that turned out to be absolutely wrong. Mass consensus on incorrect theories has often impeded vital research, delayed the development of cures or effective therapies for many conditions, and cost countless lives.

A number of medical protocols once deemed the standard of care have later proved to be harmful, and even deadly. For example, the 1899 edition of the *Merck Manual*, the prestigious medical text physicians worldwide regard as their bible, officially recommends poisons such as arsenic, ether, chloroform, turpentine oil, mercury, and strychnine as treatment for anemia, constipation, earaches and headaches.[183] Before modern-day doctors agreed that exposure to X-rays and other forms of radiation cause genetic damage and cancers, radiation was routinely administered for tonsillitis, acne, ringworm, and enlarged lymph and thymus glands.[184]

A Brief History of Mismanaged Epidemics

Disease	Popular Consensus	Actual Cause
Scurvy: 19th Century, England	Contagious Microbe	Malnutrition: Vitamin C deficiency
Beriberi: Late 1800s, Far East	Contagious Microbe	Malnutrition: Thiamin deficiency
Maternal Fever: 1900s, US and Europe	Non-contagious	Contagious: Doctors using unsanitary medical practices
Influenza: 1918, US and Europe	Bacteria	Virus
Pellagra: 1920s, US and Europe	Contagious	Malnutrition: Niacin deficiency
SMON: 1960s–1970s, Japan	New Virus	**Iatrogenic:** Pharmaceutical drug

DES (Diethylstilbestrol), a synthetic hormone given in the 1950s to prevent miscarriages in pregnant women was later found to cause cervical cancer and sterility in the daughters of women who used it.[185] Thalidomide, a popular sleeping aid prescribed during the same era was banned after it caused limb deformities in many babies born to women taking the drug.[186]

During the 1960s and 70s, an entire epidemic was caused by Clioquinol, a widely used prescription medicine for diarrhea. For 15 years, doctors and scientists blamed a virus for the sudden outbreak of a new intestinal disorder and gave suffering patients the very drug that was the cause of their illness.

Iatrogenic: Induced in a patient by a doctor's actions.

By the time a minority view was considered and the drug responsible for the epidemic was finally banned, thousands had died and many victims were left blind or paralyzed.[187]

The earning power of "annuity medicines"—drugs used throughout a lifetime to control symptoms—wields great influence over healthcare consensus today. To take just one example, stomach ulcers have been traditionally blamed on stress, diet or excess acid. For fifty years, doctors routinely prescribed antacid drugs for temporary relief—drugs that usually prompt the stomach to produce more acid. Surgery to remove portions of the stomach or to cut sensitive stomach nerves was the state of the art in ulcer treatment until the 1976 arrival of Tagamet, a pharmaceutical that blocks acid secretion.[188] By 1980, annual sales of Tagamet had reached $600 million, inspiring *Fortune* magazine to call it "one of the most stunningly successful products in the history of American business." In 1981, a similar drug Zantac was approved for use, and since 1988, has been the biggest selling drug in history.[189] Neither drug gets rid of ulcers which remain a chronic, but more manageable problem. In fact, profits from treating the ongoing symptoms of ulcers may be preventing access to a simple, inexpensive cure discovered more than 15 years ago: A two-week course of antibiotics that kill the H pylori bacteria responsible for 80% of ulcers. Since doctors rely on drug companies for treatment updates and continuing education, and the drug companies are not promoting the new findings, patients and healthcare practitioners remain unaware of the important breakthrough.[190]

Conventional Wisdom: Words from the Mainstream

"There is no definitive peer-reviewed scientific literature on the long term efficacy of protease inhibitors, yet it would be criminal not to use them."

Dr. Charles Carpenter, Director, International Health Institute, Brown University, *Rolling Stone*, March 6, 1997

"Important safety information: About 5% (5 in 100) of patients who take ZIAGEN have a serious allergic reaction that may result in death. IF YOU HAVE SKIN RASH OR TWO OF THE FOLLOWING SYMPTOMS, STOP TAKING ZIAGEN AND CALL YOUR DOCTOR IMMEDIATELY: fever, nausea, vomiting, diarrhea or abdominal pain, severe tiredness, achiness, or generally ill feeling...

"The most common side effects of ZIAGEN are skin rashes...fever...nausea, vomiting...diarrhea...abdominal pain...tiredness...muscle and joint pain, generally ill feeling...Most of these side effects do not cause people to stop taking ZIAGEN."

Glaxo-Wellcome ad for the anti-HIV drug ZIAGEN, March 1999

"If the virus doesn't get you, the drugs you take will."

Steve Gendin, Contributing Editor, *POZ* magazine, January 1999

"One of the major barriers to effectively treating HIV is that most people do not feel sick at the time they are offered anti-HIV medications. In fact, it is only after starting the medications that they begin to feel sick."

Dr. Lori Swick, *The Toronto Star*, September 24, 1999

"Here we are, knocking down handfuls of drugs that nobody really knows a lot about...and as research keeps coming up with newer and better medications that we also don't know very much about, we'll take them anyway. We're knocking down chemicals that are totally, completely foreign to almost everyone, including nature...but with a little luck, a positive outlook, and good nutrition, health improvement will happen."

Jennifer Jensen, RD (deceased), Nutritional advisor for the AIDS organization Being Alive, *Women Alive Newsletter*, September 1997

"Some new AIDS drugs are beginning to produce serious toxic conditions in patients: an increased prevalence of premature heart disease, a serious form of obesity known as lipodystrophy, and liver disease. What we have is a tremendous improvement over what we used to have, but we must find ways to reduce life-threatening toxicity. That's why the search for a cure for AIDS, however unlikely, should not be given up."

Dr. Joep Lange, AIDS treatment specialist,
The Globe and Mail, May 4, 1999

"Failures are occurring right and left...They aren't dying of traditionally defined AIDS illnesses. I don't know what they're dying of...but they're just wasting and dying. While we are making good guesses, they are just guesses. We don't know what we are doing."

Dr. Michael Saag, AIDS researcher, University of Alabama at Birmingham, *Esquire* magazine, April 1999

"When there wasn't effective [AIDS] treatment, money being wasted didn't matter so much."

Michael Weinstein, founder of the $45 million nonprofit AIDS organization AIDS Health Care Foundation, *The Wall Street Journal*, December 20, 1996

"If the spread of HIV continues, by 2001 there could be ten billion people infected hypothetically...however the population of the world is only five billion. Could we be facing the threat of extinction during our lifetime?"

Theresa Crenshaw, President's AIDS Commission, 1987,
SPIN magazine, June 1995

"Remember the APLA position: HIV is a necessary but not sufficient cause of AIDS."

Lee Klosinski, Education Division, AIDS Project Los Angeles, memo to Speaker's Bureau volunteers, April 1993

"Question for Class Discussion: You have just read some of the evidence for and against HIV being the cause of AIDS. Assuming you agree with the vast majority of HIV/AIDS investigators worldwide, that HIV does cause AIDS, do you think there comes a time at which dissenters forfeit their right to make claims on other people's time and trouble by the poverty of their arguments and by the wasted effort and exasperation they have caused?"

AIDS Update 1999, a college textbook by Gerald J. Stein, PhD, Prentice Hall Inc.

"We don't know what the long-term effects of AZT use during pregnancy might be, but so far we have seen virtually no adverse effects in the short term...Not one single tumor. Not one...I mean [the children] have cancers, lymphomas, and other problems like that...but there's no reason to link those cancers to AZT."

Dr. Ellen Cooper, Principal researcher of the Women and Infants Transmission Study, *Mothering* magazine, September/October 1998

"I know we've seen some webbed fingers...but these birth defects are cosmetic and don't interfere with life."

Mary Caffrey, Nurse-practitioner, Pediatric Division of the University of San Diego Medical Center, on AZT-generated birth defects, *Zenger's*, Issue 63, September 1999

"We are still very confused about the mechanisms that lead to CD4 T cell depletion, but at least now we are confused at a higher level of understanding."

Dr. Paul Johnson, Harvard Medical School, *Science* magazine, May 1997

"Sometimes we virologists have a virus in search of a disease."

Dr. Robert Gallo, *Virus Hunting*, Basic Books, 1991

"An AIDS vaccine should be ready for testing in about two years."

Margaret Heckler, Head of Health and Human Services, April 24, 1984

"Newark and New Jersey have begun casting their nets for test subjects for the world's first full-scale clinical trials of an AIDS vaccine. AIDSVax is a genetically engineered drug...that triggers [HIV] antibodies that may enable a person to better protect himself as soon as he is exposed to the real virus, before the immune system is devastated. Dr. Krim of AmFar said 'AIDSVax is worth a try. And even if it is ineffective, it will be a good rehearsal on how to recruit for and test other vaccines.'"

The New York Times, June 8, 1999

"The patients who have done the best are those who have lived long enough to realize that my previous advice was incorrect."

Brian Gazzard, MD lecturing at the 12th World AIDS Conference, Geneva, Switzerland, 1998

If It's Not HIV, What Can Cause AIDS?

Contrary to popular belief, HIV is not necessary to explain acquired immune deficiency and the illnesses associated with AIDS. To understand why this is so, it is first necessary to understand what AIDS is. AIDS is not a new disease or illness; it is a new name or designation for 29 previously known diseases and conditions. As the NIH states in its comprehensive report on AIDS, "the designation 'AIDS' is a surveillance tool."[191] Since 1981, the surveillance tool AIDS has been used to track and record familiar diseases when they appear in people who have tested positive for antibodies associated with HIV.

The AIDS virus hypothesis supposes that the health problems renamed AIDS develop as a result of infection with HIV; that the virus somehow disables the body's defense system that protects against opportunistic illness, allowing the development of one or more of 29 diseases—such as yeast infection, certain cancers, pneumonia, salmonella, diarrhea, or tuberculosis—which are then diagnosed as AIDS. However, every AIDS indicator disease occurs among people who test HIV negative—none are exclusive to those who test positive—and all AIDS diseases existed before the adoption of the name "AIDS."

Prior to the designation AIDS, these 29 diseases were not thought to have a single, common cause. In fact, all have recognized causes and treatments that are unrelated to HIV. For example, yeast infection is a widespread problem due to an imbalance of natural bacteria. The yeast infections that occur in people who test HIV positive and in people who test HIV negative are caused by the same imbalance of natural bacteria. All the opportunistic illnesses called AIDS have various, medically proven causes that do not involve HIV.

Immune deficiency can be acquired by several risk factors that are not infectious or transmitted through blood or blood products. The following factors are widely recognized causes of immune suppression, compromised health, and opportunistic infections, as documented in the medical literature for more than 70 years. Chronic, habitual and multiple exposures to these risks can cause the group of symptoms called AIDS.[192] In fact, there is no case of AIDS described in the medical literature without one or more of these health risk factors.[193]

Physical Risk Factors

These risks include malnutrition and chronic lack of sleep. In 1985, orthodox AIDS researcher and director of NIAID, Dr. Anthony Fauci declared that malnutrition was the most prevalent cause of immune deficiency diseases throughout the world, particularly in developing regions such as Africa where common illnesses like measles run rampant and take millions of lives.[194]

The medical literature notes that malnutrition and infection are invariably linked, as one condition aggravates the other. Hunger and **endemic** disease

Endemic: A medical term applied to a disease or disorder that is constantly present in a particular region or in a specific group of people.

are familiar problems in those countries around the globe thought to be under siege from AIDS. Intrauterine malnutrition occurs when expectant mothers are improperly nourished, and can result in prolonged, sometimes lifelong, immune suppression.[195]

Poverty, crowded living conditions and unclean water promote endemic disease and compromised health. The populations in many developing regions of the world are devastated by rampant infections with common microbes that pose little or no health threat to people in industrialized nations.

Infections due to malnutrition immunodeficiency are the world's leading causes of infant and child death.[195] Among citizens of industrialized nations, subclinical malnutrition, rather than starvation leads to compromised immune function, especially when combined with chronic lack of sleep.[196] People who make habitual and prolonged use of certain drugs like methamphetamines, heroin and crack cocaine often suffer from malnutrition and chronic lack of sleep.

Chemical Risk Factors

Immune-compromising chemicals include pharmaceutical drugs such as AZT and other **cancer chemotherapy** compounds, protease inhibitors, antibiotics and steroids, and recreational drugs such as cocaine, crack, heroin, nitrites (poppers), and methamphetamines (crystal, speed).

Chemotherapy targets and destroys the bone marrow cells from which all immune cells derive. They also kill fully formed immune cells in addition to killing B cells and red blood cells.[196,197] Chemotherapy destroys the digestive system by killing the cells that compose the inner lining of the digestive tract which interferes with the body's ability to absorb and digest nutrients, causing malnutrition. Even when used very briefly, chemotherapy suppresses normal immune function, increases susceptibility to a variety of opportunistic infections, and can cause life-threatening anemia and diarrhea. AZT, ddI, ddC, D4T and 3TC are all chemotherapy compounds used as antiviral AIDS treatments.

There are many pharmaceutical drugs known to suppress the immune system, particularly when used for prolonged periods of time. Protease inhibitors cause impaired liver function and liver failure (the liver removes disease-causing toxins from the body) in addition to kidney failure, dangerously high cholesterol levels, diarrhea and other health-compromising effects. Steroids are a known cause of immune deficiency often prescribed to AIDS patients to counteract the muscle wasting caused by AZT.[198] Antibiotics, especially when used habitually, can cause yeast infection and diarrhea, two conditions that can lead to malnutrition.[199] Septra and Bactrim are sulfonamide antibiotics commonly prescribed for continuous, prophylactic or preventative use by HIV positives. These drugs are leftover from the days before penicillin; they do not

Cancer chemotherapy: Drugs used to treat cancer. Most anticancer drugs are cytotoxic (kill or damage cells). Others are synthetic forms of hormones. All anticancer drugs prevent cells from growing and dividing. Some work by damaging the cell's DNA; others block the chemical processes in the cell necessary for growth. Side effects of treatment include nausea, vomiting, and life-threatening diarrhea. By altering the rate at which cells grow and divide, anticancer drugs reduce the number of blood cells produced by the bone marrow, causing anemia and increased susceptibility to infection.

target invading microbes as narrowly as modern antibiotics and are notorious for their side effects.[200] Both cause nausea, diarrhea, vomiting, anorexia, bone marrow destruction, rashes, fever, hepatitis, and anemia by interfering with the production of red blood cells.[201]

The immunosuppressive effects of recreational drug abuse are well-documented in medical literature dating back to the turn of the century. They include pneumonias, mouth sores, fevers, **endocarditis**, bacterial infections and night sweats—all conditions now associated with AIDS.[202] Amphetamine drugs suppress the appetite, causing chronic users to suffer from malnutrition. Many habitual users of heroin and crack do not provide themselves with adequate food, sleep, shelter and healthcare.

Prolonged exposure to common chemical toxins such as insecticides and herbicides can also impair immune function.[203]

Biological Risk Factors

These risks include multiple exposures to and/or chronic infections with syphilis, gonorrhea, chlamydia and other venereal diseases, hepatitis, tuberculosis, malaria, fungal diseases, amoebas and parasites such as giardia, bacterial infections such as staph and E coli, chronic bowel infections, blood transfusions, and the use of blood products. In addition to the damaging effects of recurrent infections, many of the pharmaceuticals used as treatment have adverse effects on immune function.

Factor VIII (the blood clotting agent used by hemophiliacs) and blood transfusions are immune suppressive and leave patients vulnerable to infection.[204] Due to the serious conditions for which transfusions are necessary and the deleterious effects they have on the immune system, half of all HIV negative transfusion recipients die within a year of receiving a transfusion.[204]

Psychological Risk Factors

Chronic anxiety, panic, stress and depression have been shown to compromise health, damage immune function, and result in symptoms identical to AIDS.[205] Mental stress provokes production of the hormone cortisol; excessive cortisol causes rapid and dramatic reductions in T cells, a condition known as lymphocytopenia. Within minutes, stress induces cortisol levels to increase as much as 20-fold. High levels of cortisol can eventually cause what medical texts describe as "significant atrophy of all the lymphoid tissue throughout the body" which may lead to "fulminating infection and death from diseases that would otherwise not be lethal."[206]

A profound fear of AIDS is enough to cause even people who repeatedly test HIV negative to develop physical symptoms of AIDS.[207] Termed "AIDS-phobia," this condition is characterized by weight loss, wasting, reduced T cell counts and other signs considered indicative of AIDS, and typically follows intimate contact with people who sufferers believe may be HIV positive.

Endocarditis: Inflammation of the internal lining of the heart.

Beliefs and expectations are well-known to manifest in the physical body. The life-altering influence of beliefs was detailed dramatically in 1942 by Dr. Walter B. Cannon in his accounts of a phenomenon he called "voodoo death," a form of capital punishment practiced among certain Aboriginal tribes. Cannon reported that shaman, tribal medical authorities thought to possess special powers, were able to kill errant tribe members by simply pointing at them with a bone. Convinced of the shaman's ability to invoke a lethal curse, the people pointed at died within a matter of hours or days.[208]

In modern medicine, the power of expectation is a commonly accepted fact known as the "placebo effect." Placebos are inert chemical substances disguised as active preparations and given to patients in place of drugs. The health benefits gained from a placebo occur because the person taking it expects a positive effect. Since the benefits of any drug may be due in part to this placebo effect, most new drugs are tested against a placebo preparation.[209]

A recent study conducted at the University of Toronto demonstrated the profound physiological effects of expectation with regard to placebos. Researchers found that cardiac patients who strictly adhered to a placebo treatment regimen lived longer than patients who did not take their placebo regularly. In summarizing the study, lead researcher Dr. Paul Dorian noted, "What you believe has an important influence on your outcome."[210]

How These Risk Factors Apply to All AIDS Groups

There is not one case of AIDS described in the medical literature that does not include one or more immune-destroying health risk factors. There is no case of AIDS documented in a person whose sole risk is exposure to HIV. Every case of AIDS involves factors known to damage the immune system and leave a person vulnerable to debilitating infection and deadly illness.[211]

Men Who Have Sex With Men

Well-documented causes of immune dysfunction can explain AIDS illnesses among men who have sex with men although none of these causes are unique to this risk group or can be generalized to include all gay men. In fact, focusing attention on certain sexual practices rather than recognized health risks obscures our understanding of immune suppression and limits approaches to preventing and resolving AIDS.

Nitrites, more commonly known as poppers, are immune-suppressive, carcinogenic drugs chronically used by some gay men. At one time, 95% of gay men in major urban areas like Los Angeles, New York and San Francisco reported using poppers.[212] Nitrite use correlates with Kaposi's Sarcoma (KS) and non-Hodgkin's lymphoma, two AIDS-defining cancers found almost exclusively in this risk group.[213] There are several studies that further strengthen the correlation between poppers and KS by documenting KS in HIV negative gay men who use poppers.[213] KS is hardly ever found among members of any other CDC risk group or among women with AIDS, and is never diagnosed in children or infants with AIDS.[213] In 1981 when AIDS was first identified, half of all AIDS diagnoses were for KS. As popper use has diminished, so has KS which since 1993 has accounted for less than 5% of all new AIDS cases.[214]

In the only studies that asked gay men with AIDS about recreational drugs, 93% to 100% of participants acknowledged using cocaine, crack cocaine, poppers, heroin, ecstasy, methamphetamines like speed and crystal, and/or Special K (an animal tranquilizer).[215]

Combinations of parasitic infections that include amebiasis and giardiasis along with rectal infections, syphilis, and gonorrhea can result in acute diarrhea which in turn causes malabsorption and malnutrition, or wasting.[216] This collection of infections and resultant problems was commonly known as Gay Bowel Syndrome in the years before AIDS.[216] The CDC reports that 20% to 50% of all gay men in major US cities have been treated, often repeatedly, for intestinal parasites using immune suppressive pharmaceutical drugs.[217] Antibiotic treatments for recurrent venereal infections are immune suppressive, as is the practice of using these antibiotics on a regular basis as a prevention. Steroids are another immune damaging drug frequently prescribed to offset the wasting caused by diarrhea and malabsorption.[217]

Campaigns that encourage HIV testing, the consuming of toxic AIDS drugs, and living in fear of AIDS are primarily directed at the gay community. Many gay magazines may have up to half of their commercial advertising devoted to AIDS-related promotions.[218] Such constant emphasis on AIDS gives rise to the notion of the inevitability of AIDS, a belief which can evoke chronic terror, despair and hopelessness—psychological risk factors known to impair immunity and compromise health.

The chance of registering false positive on an HIV test is greater for people with high levels of non-HIV antibodies and microbes in their blood. Antibodies produced in response to the particular microbial and viral infections frequently found in some gay men are documented causes of false positive HIV test results.[218]

For people who test HIV positive, the drugs prescribed as preventative treatments for opportunistic AIDS-defining infections become harmful and even deadly when used on a daily, continuous basis. Bactrim and Septra, for example, are powerful sulfonamide antibiotics that kill digestive flora and cause anemia and bone marrow destruction. The anti-HIV drugs AZT, ddI, D4T, ddC and 3TC are all highly toxic chemotherapies that destroy the immune and digestive systems, in addition to causing five of the 29 official AIDS-defining illnesses.[219] Two 1993 studies conducted in the US and Canada found that every one of several hundred gay men with AIDS had a history of significant recreational drug and/or AIDS drug use.[220]

Identifying this risk group as people who engage in habitual, prolonged use of recreational and/or pharmaceutical drugs, have chronic exposure to a multitude of infectious microbes, who suffer from chronic malnourishment and/or chronic fear of HIV and AIDS provides a more appropriate and comprehensive explanation of immune suppression that invites many possibilities for prevention and resolution.

Injection Drug Users

Members of this risk group account for 35% of all diagnosed AIDS cases, while another 4% of people diagnosed with AIDS cite heterosexual contact with injection drug users as their sole risk. However, the majority of people who initially claim intimate contact with IV drug users as their only risk later acknowledge taking drugs themselves.[221]

Considering only injection drug use as a high risk activity for AIDS disregards the immune suppressive effects brought about by habitual use of non-injected street drugs as well as the many health-compromising factors that can accompany the regular, long-term use of illicit chemicals. The emphasis on sharing needles over the damaging effects of the narcotics injected with the needles distorts our view of immune dysfunction and prevents application of practical solutions to the health problems common to this risk group.

Drug Diseases Diagnosed Before the AIDS Era in HIV-Free Drug Users[222]

	Disease	Drug Used			
		Cocaine	*Heroin*	*Nitrites*	*Amphetamines*
AIDS Defining Diseases	Immunodeficiency[1c]	✔	✔	✔	✔
AIDS Defining Diseases	Kaposi's sarcoma[2c]			✔	
AIDS Defining Diseases	Candidiasis[3c]	✔	✔		
AIDS Defining Diseases	Pneumonia[4c]	✔	✔	✔	
AIDS Defining Diseases	Lymphadenopathy[5c]	✔	✔		
AIDS Defining Diseases	Tuberculosis[6c]	✔	✔		
AIDS Defining Diseases	Weight loss[7c]	✔	✔		
AIDS Defining Diseases	Dementia, encephalopathy[8c]	✔	✔		
AIDS Defining Diseases	Diarrhea[9c]	✔	✔		
AIDS Defining Diseases	Fever[10c]	✔	✔		
	Spontaneous abortion, premature birth, congenital abnormalities[11c]	✔	✔		
	Night sweats[12c]	✔	✔		
	Impotence[13c]	✔	✔		
	Severe atherosclerosis[14c]				✔
	Tooth loss, cavities[15c]	✔	✔		
	Dermatitis[16c]	✔	✔		
	Hepatitis[17c]	✔	✔		
	Epileptic seizures[18c]	✔	✔		
	Endocarditis[19c]	✔	✔		
	Bronchitis[20c]	✔	✔		

Prolonged, habitual consumption of drugs such as heroin, crack, speed, and cocaine, whether taken by injection or other means, is well-known to disable immune function. Chronic use of these drugs is documented to bring about many conditions synonymous with AIDS including pneumonias, tuberculosis, mouth sores, fevers, night sweats, bacterial infections, and endocarditis. Malnutrition—the number one cause of immune deficiency diseases worldwide—and multiple infections are frequent side effects of habitual injection drug use, and are factors that suppress immunity.

Antibodies generated in response to the multiple infections and chemical toxins typical of chronic drug use can cause false positive readings on HIV tests. Positive test results most frequently lead to ongoing treatment with various immune suppressive antibiotics and chemotherapy drugs, and to a sense of hopelessness and profound despair.

A more compassionate and inclusive way to portray this diverse group is as people who engage in habitual, prolonged use of recreational drugs, have chronic exposure to a multitude of infectious microbes and toxins through septic syringes or septic living conditions; who suffer from chronic malnourishment, lack of adequate sleep, the immune suppressive effects of AIDS drugs, and/or the chronic despair that follows an HIV positive or AIDS diagnosis. The immune deficiency diseases caused by these multiple and variant factors can be resolved with treatments that do not involve toxic anti-HIV drugs and long-term use of powerful antibiotics.

Transfusion Recipients and Hemophiliacs

Hemophiliacs and blood transfusion recipients together make up 2% of adult AIDS cases in the US. As noted previously, Factor VIII, the blood clotting treatment used by hemophiliacs, is itself immune suppressive. Hemophilia is a life-threatening condition in people with or without an HIV positive diagnosis. Ryan White, the young HIV positive hemophiliac who became famous as an AIDS victim, actually died of common complications attributed to hemophilia (internal bleeding and liver failure), not of illnesses that define AIDS.[223]

Blood transfusions suppress the immune system. Medical experts note that higher amounts of blood transfusions among hospitalized patients correlate with higher death rates. The authors of one recent study on transfusions specifically mention that the immune suppressive effects of transfusions leave recipients vulnerable to deadly opportunistic infection.[224]

Factor VIII and blood transfusions can cause positive results on HIV antibody tests in persons never exposed to HIV by triggering the production of antibodies that react with the nonspecific proteins used in the HIV antibody test. Once a person has tested positive, they are subject to immune suppressive drug treatment regimens, and the terror of developing AIDS.

Members of these risk groups can be more accurately described as people with serious preexisting health challenges, critical or chronic exposure to immune suppressive blood products and toxic AIDS drugs, and/or who are affected by the chronic despair of a fatal diagnosis. Based on this view, immune compromising anti-HIV chemotherapy and continuous antibiotic treatments would compound preexisting health problems, rather than resolve them.

Heterosexual Contact

Six percent of Americans diagnosed with AIDS cite heterosexual contact as their sole AIDS risk. However, upon further investigation, 60% to 99% of these people are reclassified as injection drug users and/or men who have sex with men, groups with identifiable health risks documented to cause immune dysfunction.[225] As previously noted, people diagnosed with AIDS voluntarily select a risk group from among six categories determined by the CDC which limits health risks to possible exposure to HIV through sex or blood.

The damage caused by AIDS chemotherapy and the acceptance of a fatal diagnosis are sufficient to bring about serious illness and even death in people with no other risk factors.

Members of this group may be better described as people with no health risk factors acknowledged by the CDC who, because of their positive HIV status, regularly consume chemotherapy and/or engage in continuous treatment with antibiotics and other immune suppressive pharmaceutical drugs, and/or suffer from the chronic panic and hopelessness of a fatal diagnosis.

Adolescents, Children and Infants

Although teenagers and children are not a specific AIDS risk group, cases of AIDS among young people, however rare, are a matter of great concern. The fact that babies are diagnosed with AIDS has been used as an argument against non-HIV explanations for AIDS illnesses. Despite widely held beliefs, the majority of AIDS cases that occur among children and adolescents can be explained by the same causes of immune suppression prevalent in adults with AIDS.

In 1998, new AIDS cases among this country's 26 million teens totaled 293; of these, 229 offered information which placed them in the two primary CDC defined AIDS risk groups for adults.[226]

Over 80% of the mothers of babies diagnosed with AIDS voluntarily acknowledge using injection drugs during pregnancy, a practice which almost universally results in intrauterine malnutrition. The remaining cases of AIDS in infants and children may be due to the immune suppressive medical treatments given in response to an HIV positive test result, or to the same factors that cause HIV negative babies to suffer from pneumonia, bacterial infections, and immune disorders. In 1998, new AIDS cases in children age 13 and under totaled 382.[227]

Residents of Developing Nations

In stark contrast to the US and Europe, AIDS cases in developing areas of the world are found almost exclusively among non-drug using heterosexuals.[228] Mainstream AIDS experts offer no plausible reason why AIDS would spread primarily through drug-free heterosexual contact only outside the US and Europe.

A coherent explanation for AIDS cases in developing areas of the world is the well-known health risks shared by these countries—widespread poverty and malnutrition; lack of clean water, a regular food supply, and sanitary living conditions; limited access to medical care; endemic diseases such as tuberculosis, malaria, and parasitic infections that manifest in conditions identical to AIDS; and the practice of diagnosing AIDS based on a nonspecific set of clinical symptoms.

Although HIV tests are not required for an AIDS diagnosis in many parts of the world, widespread exposure to hepatitis, tuberculosis, leprosy, malaria and other conditions are more than sufficient to account for positive results on the nonspecific HIV antibody tests.[229]

Resolving the immune suppressive conditions caused by poverty and malnutrition provides a means to alleviate the suffering of many people in developing nations who are currently counted and treated as victims of AIDS.

When considering non-HIV explanations for AIDS, consider that:

- AIDS is a collection of familiar illnesses, not a disease.
- Since 1993, more than half of all new AIDS diagnoses in the US are given to people who are not ill. In 1997, two-thirds of Americans diagnosed with AIDS had no symptoms or illness.*
- Acquired immune deficiency predates the creation of the category "AIDS" and has numerous, well-documented causes.
- There are no AIDS cases noted in the medical literature in which exposure to HIV has proved to be the sole health risk factor.
- There are well-documented causes for every AIDS disease that do not involve HIV, and all illnesses now called AIDS occur in the absence of HIV.
- HIV tests do not test for the actual virus, but for antiviral proteins or genetic material that are not specific to HIV.
- The chance of a positive reaction on a nonspecific HIV antibody test increases proportionately with the level of other antibodies and microbes found in the blood.
- Five of the six AIDS risk groups defined by the CDC have health risk factors that involve multiple, chronic exposure to viruses, bacteria and other antigens known to produce antibodies identical to those associated with HIV.
- Once a person has tested HIV antibody positive, chemotherapy and other immune suppressing chemicals are almost always prescribed for treatment or prevention of AIDS.
- Alternative explanations for AIDS provide opportunities for effective AIDS prevention and for using practical, nontoxic approaches to resolving AIDS.

* 1997 was the last year that the CDC provided information on how many AIDS cases were diagnosed in people who are not sick.

Incorrect Information about HIV and AIDS Costs Lives

Can you imagine receiving a fatal diagnosis without being told the diagnosis is based on an unproven idea and an uncertain test? Being instructed to take powerful, experimental drugs without being told these drugs compromise health, destroy functions necessary to sustain life, and were approved for use without adequate testing? Being informed that you have, or should expect, deadly illnesses without being told that these same illnesses are not considered fatal when they occur in "normal" people?

For anyone who tests HIV positive, getting all the facts is a matter of life and death. The important decisions a person makes should be based on thorough, verifiable data. All of us need and have the right to receive honest and complete information about HIV and AIDS.

Almost every AIDS organization in the country offers free instruction for people who test HIV positive. Standard information includes how to prepare a will, how to collect disability, health insurance, and public benefits, what drugs and tests to take, and which diseases to anticipate—all based on the assumption that HIV positives are or will be ill and do not have long to live.

Information on AIDS that is free from bias, that accurately describes tests and drugs, and offers facts that support a will to live, participate in society, and cultivate a healthy future are rarely, if ever mentioned. Some AIDS groups even lobby to limit public access to data that undermine their dire presentations of HIV and AIDS.

For many people handed an HIV positive diagnosis, these brief pages provide their first awareness that a normal, healthy life is not something they can only hope for, but something they can choose to achieve. Unfortunately for most people who test positive, the AIDS education they receive portrays their choices as being limited to toxic drug therapy or devastating illness, and encourages chronic fear, sadness, and resignation to an early death.

There are thousands of HIV positives who lead healthy lives without toxic AIDS drugs. What they have in common is not some unique, mysterious gene or a weakened strain of the virus, but an open-minded approach to information, an understanding of basic principles of medicine and science, and the knowledge that the responsibility for their well-being is ultimately their own. For more information on their lives, please see *The Other Side of AIDS* on page 94.

This book examines only a portion of the growing body of scientific, medical and epidemiological evidence that refutes popularly accepted ideas about HIV and AIDS. Readers are strongly encouraged to conduct further research and use the resources offered here.

Incorrect Ideas about HIV and AIDS Cost Us All

To the degree that we allow unfounded ideas about HIV and AIDS to determine our actions, influence our choices, dictate our public policies, or define our world view, we are all victims of AIDS.

Since the 1984 announcement that HIV causes AIDS, all AIDS research has been based on the hypothesis that HIV, an inexplicably lethal new virus, is responsible for a group of previously known, disconnected diseases renamed AIDS. Setting the focus of all AIDS efforts on HIV, a virus that strains the rules of biology, epidemiology and logic, has rendered humankind few, if any, beneficial results.

The lives of over 400,000 Americans have been given to the notion that HIV is the only possible cause of AIDS, and that toxic drugs offer the only possible prevention, treatment, or hope for a cure. Many more lives have been forever altered by a positive result on a non-standardized test for harmless antibodies that may or may not be associated with HIV.

More than $50 billion in federal AIDS funding has provided no significant understanding of HIV, has produced no safe and effective therapies, and has not brought us any closer to ending AIDS. Instead, we have constructed a powerful AIDS establishment that regulates our news, limits our access to information, and demands an ever greater allocation of our resources and support. Rather than helping to resolve AIDS, we have funded the growth of multi-billion dollar industries, institutions and organizations that depend on AIDS and on our continued devotion to the narrow and unproductive HIV hypothesis.

Objective Examination of HIV and AIDS is Fundamental to Progress.

To understand and solve AIDS, it is necessary to investigate all legitimate scientific data, even when such information challenges our present understanding and perceptions. Progress in any area depends on the ability to engage in an unbiased evaluation of facts, to raise critical questions and to conduct an objective search for meaningful answers.

Silence = Death...Of People, Ideas and Progress

"There is classical science—the way it's supposed to work—and then there's religion. I regained my sanity when I realized that AIDS science was a religious discourse. The one thing I will go to my grave not understanding is why everyone was so quick to accept everything the government said as truth. Especially the central myth: The cause of AIDS is known. What in the world made activists accept that—on the basis of a press conference, no less?

"My only theory is that AIDS requires the daily management of massive amounts of uncertainty, and people cling to any certainty they can find. Even if it's false."

Michael Callen, author, AIDS activist (deceased),
Genre magazine, February/March, 1994

"Most HIV trials are useless rubbish. Research scientists [outside AIDS research] laugh at us. To them a good sample size is 30,000 people. We do studies with 1,500 people and think that's wonderful when the actual number of relevant patients is sometimes so small, you cannot rule out chance as the reason for the results you get. It is also unethical to run trials of drugs in places like Malaysia with only 30 people involved and then try to justify these flawed trials because some people got access to drugs who otherwise would have had nothing."

Kevin Frost, Manager of Research Programs for the American Foundation for AIDS Research (AmFAR), *Positive Nation*, September 1998

"The story of AIDS is deeply connected with the vicissitudes of the theory that viruses cause cancer and the failure of the cancer research program. Michael Verney-Elliot put it most acidly when he said: 'From the people who didn't bring you the virus that causes cancer, it's the virus that doesn't cause AIDS.'"

Jad Adams, Author, *The HIV Myth*, 1989

"AIDS is not another disease, it is the most metaphorical disease in history. It is the ultimate triumph of politics over science."

Michael Fumento, Author, *The Myth of Heterosexual AIDS*, 1990

"Perhaps I'd feel different about it if I thought people were dying from AIDS. But I don't. I think they're dying from bad medicine, bad drugs, bad attitudes. There is nothing I want from 'Big Daddy'—I don't want his medicines, his laws, his approval."

Gavin Dillard, Author, *In the Flesh*, HIV positive since 1985, *San Francisco Frontiers*, May 20, 1999

"In the September 4 issue of the *Journal of the American Medical Association*, the CDC announced that a diagnosis of AIDS no longer requires an HIV test. The government now considers you an AIDS carrier if you suffer from any of the maladies on its new list of diseases indicative of AIDS, including such relatively common infections as herpes simplex, tuberculosis, Salmonellosis and the shockingly broad category 'other bacterial infections.' This broad definition will lead to countless new AIDS diagnoses—whether or not the person actually has AIDS. A major problem with the new AIDS definition is that it ignores the many environmental causes of immune suppression. Exposure to toxins, alcoholism, heavy drug use or heavy antibiotic use all can cause onset of the list of 'diseases' indicative of AIDS. The CDC itself conceded in a stunning remark near the end of the *JAMA* article that the new AIDS ground rules are highly suspect. 'The diagnostic criteria accepted by the AIDS surveillance case definition should not be interpreted as the standard of good medical practice,' warned the CDC."

Los Angeles Weekly, December 18, 1987

"The real trick is to get off the medication. I felt I was losing quality of life..."

Greg Louganis, HIV positive Olympic Gold Medalist, *The State*, April 15, 1997

"It's not even probable, let alone scientifically proven, that HIV causes AIDS. If there is evidence that HIV causes AIDS, there should be scientific documents which either singly or collectively demonstrate that fact, at least with a high probability. There are no such documents."

Dr. Kary Mullis, Nobel Laureate,
HIV not Guilty, October 5, 1996

"If you think a virus is the cause of AIDS, do a control without it. To do a control is the first thing you teach undergraduates. But it hasn't been done. The epidemiology of AIDS is a pile of anecdotal stories selected to fit the virus-AIDS hypothesis. People don't bother to check the details of popular dogma or consensus views."

Dr. Peter Duesberg, *Do You Think HIV Causes AIDS?*,
Scientists for Legitimacy in Science, 1995

"Beware the scientist who believes that mainstream research thinking on any public health issue is equivalent to truth. Or the scientist who bullies or ridicules other scientists because they oppose the prevailing view. This is a person who has become what I would call a propagandist and should not be trusted.

"I have worked as a medical science reporter for 30 years. I've interviewed thousands of scientists for newspaper and magazine stories, radio and television productions, and books. I've met scientists who at least try to keep an open and fair mind on scientific issues. I have also met many propagandists who think they're scientists. In all the time I've worked as a journalist, I've never come across a nastier group of people to interview than those propagandists who work in HIV research."

Nicholas Regush, Medical Science Reporter, Second Opinion,
ABCNews.com, September 29, 1999

"As a scientist who has studied AIDS for 16 years, I have determined that AIDS has little to do with science and is not even primarily a medical issue. AIDS is a sociological phenomenon held together by fear, creating a kind of medical McCarthyism that has transgressed and collapsed all the rules of science, and has imposed a brew of belief and pseudoscience on a vulnerable public."

Dr. David Rasnick, Designer of Protease Inhibitors,
SPIN magazine, June 1997

"Considering there is little scientific proof of the exact linkage of HIV and AIDS, is it ethical to prescribe AZT, a toxic chain terminator of DNA developed 30 years ago as cancer chemotherapy, to 150,000 Americans—among them pregnant women and newborn babies—as an anti-HIV drug?"

Rep. Gil Gutknecht (R-MN), US House of Representatives,
Letter to NIAID Director Dr. Anthony Fauci, March 14, 1995

If You Have Tested Positive...

Although a diagnosis of HIV positive is widely considered evidence of infection with a lethal virus, you have the right to question this diagnosis and to determine what testing HIV positive will mean to you. Your health is ultimately your responsibility, and with the current state of orthodox AIDS information and treatments, it is especially important that you become your own health advocate. You can start by building a solid foundation of knowledge upon which to base important choices regarding the rest of your life. Connecting with, or creating a support network of well-informed peers and health professionals can make it easier for you to put fear and outside pressure into perspective, cultivate wellness, and stay focused on the facts.

Be aware that your physical health is greatly influenced by what you accept as true about HIV and AIDS. Beliefs can be as potent as any drug or microbe, and living in terror of HIV and AIDS is guaranteed to produce devastating physiological effects. To the degree that it is possible, stay calm, hold a picture of health in your mind, and surround yourself with life-affirming influences while you work to replace detrimental beliefs and unfounded fears with factual information.

For everyone who receives a positive test result, HIV is the beginning of a journey. You have the right and the ability to choose what paths you will take on your journey. Remember that there is another side to popular news and information about HIV and AIDS.

Keep in mind these helpful facts about testing HIV positive:

- Viral antibodies alone do not cause or predict illness; in fact, they are an indication of a normal, healthy immune response and provide protection from disease. There is no evidence to indicate that HIV antibodies differ in any way from helpful, protective antibodies.
- Since HIV antigens cross-react with antibodies produced in response to numerous diseases and microbes commonly found in normal, healthy people, a positive HIV test result does not confirm past exposure to HIV.
- Since HIV antibody tests have never been calibrated against virus isolation, their true accuracy has never been established which means that there is no substantiation for the claim that testing HIV positive indicates a present infection with HIV.
- People in AIDS risks groups are at high risk for testing false positive on HIV antibody tests. Injection drug users, hemophiliacs, blood transfusion recipients, people from areas of the world where malaria, hepatitis, tuberculosis, leprosy and parasitic infections are endemic, and certain gay men have been exposed to many foreign antigens and infectious agents documented to give false positive results on HIV tests.

- Actual HIV is never directly detected in people who test positive on the antibody tests.
- Viral load tests cannot diagnose illness, measure HIV infection or determine state of health. Viral load tests do not detect actual virus and are not approved by the FDA for diagnostic use. As the manufacturers' own literature states, the test "is not intended to be used to confirm the presence of HIV..."
- No type of viral load test has ever been verified by virus isolation.
- In the only published study that compares viral load results against the finding of HIV by co-culture, more than half of people with detectable levels of viral load had zero virus.[230]
- It is possible to receive an AIDS diagnosis even though you are not ill or suffering from any symptoms of immune suppression.

It is important to note that although you may choose to live without regard to your HIV status, there are legal ramifications to testing HIV positive that cannot be ignored. As unfair and misguided as these regulations may be, they do exist. At present, 32 states in America have criminal statutes on "transmission of HIV" and 17 of these make it a felony crime for a person who has tested HIV positive to engage in many forms of sexual activity, including sexual intercourse. In some states, the informed consent of a sexual partner is not allowed as an affirmative defense; in other states an affirmative defense requires that the person who tests HIV positive use a condom. One state makes it illegal for anyone who tests positive to marry. For a complete list of state criminal statutes on HIV, please send a self-addressed stamped envelope to The American Foundation for AIDS Alternatives.

If You Also Face Health Challenges

The information presented in this book disputes HIV as the cause of a growing list of familiar diseases that have been officially categorized as or are popularly associated with AIDS. This challenge to the HIV hypothesis should not be interpreted as an excuse to ignore symptoms of illness, or to engage in practices known to compromise well-being.

As with any other health issue, important decisions regarding treatment options are your responsibility. Most people find that choices become clearer and easier when they are based on a thorough evaluation of facts and a wide spectrum of information.

Working with health practitioners who will help you address your actual problems, rather than focusing on the notion of HIV as the problem, is essential to real recovery. Seek out those who will regard you as a unique human being in possession of your natural ability to heal; avoid anyone who defines you by your HIV status, who believes that wellness is beyond your capability or views your health crisis through the narrow and distorted lens of HIV.

Keep in mind that the immune system is not one specific system but is the synergistic interaction of all our functioning systems and involves every organ in the body. When these systems are operating at favorable levels, we enjoy good health. Illnesses arise when one or more of these systems becomes weak, damaged, overburdened, or dysfunctional. Health is a condition of optimal well-being, the soundness of body and mind.

Although pharmaceutical treatments can be helpful and even lifesaving in certain circumstances, none are able to create or regenerate good health. Pharmaceuticals can kill microbes, quell pain, destroy cells, and suppress, incite, or replace bodily functions. In general, drugs mask the symptoms of disease rather than resolving the root cause. There is no medicine that can create good health, and no chemical or natural compound that can restore immunity. Good health is a process that requires your active participation.

There are many methods of recovery that are based on assisting the body's natural ability to heal. Some alternatives to the health-compromising drug treatments that are the primary tool of Western medicine are briefly described in *Options for Healing and Wellness* on page 69. A resource guide for further study on various approaches to health and recovery is also included in this section.

Be persistent until you find the method(s) that work for you. Be prepared to explore other options should a successful approach to one situation fail to address a recurrent or new problem. Accept the fact that just like every other human being on earth, you have the right to become ill and get better. The World Health Organization asserts that all people should have the opportunity to fulfill their genetic potential in achieving good health—this includes you.

When dealing with illness and an HIV positive diagnosis, it is necessary to remember these important facts:

- AIDS is not a disease.
- All AIDS-defining conditions occur in people who test HIV negative, none appear exclusively in those who test positive, and all existed before the adoption of the name "AIDS."
- All the illnesses called AIDS have medically recognized causes and treatments unrelated to HIV.
- The primary evidence offered in support of the hypothesis that HIV causes AIDS is a correlation between HIV and AIDS. Correlation is not proof of causation, and the appearance of a high correlation between HIV and AIDS is simply a result of the HIV-based definition of AIDS. The 29 old diseases that are used to define AIDS only count as AIDS if a person has a positive result on an HIV antibody test. In other words:

  Pneumonia + Positive HIV Test = AIDS

  Pneumonia + Negative HIV Test = Pneumonia

  Diarrhea + Positive HIV Test = AIDS

  Diarrhea + Negative HIV Test = Diarrhea

- Healthy people who test HIV positive vastly outnumber HIV positives who become sick and die. This is true in America, as well as in Africa, Haiti and other parts of the world where a large percentage of the population tests HIV positive and has limited access to medical care.[231]

- A careful review of the mainstream scientific literature reveals that HIV positives who remain AIDS-free share one essential feature: by choice or by circumstance, they do not take AIDS cocktails, antivirals or recreational drugs and do not use antibiotics on a continuous, daily basis.[232]

- Information extracted from orthodox AIDS literature confirms three common characteristics among long-term survivors: avoidance of the AIDS chemotherapy drugs AZT, ddI, ddC, d4T and 3TC; cessation of health-compromising practices upon receiving their positive diagnosis (such as recreational drug use and exposure to sexually transmitted microbes); and the introduction of health-enhancing practices such as proper nutrition, adequate rest, and regular exercise.[233]

- A study of chronically malnourished intravenous drug users who tested HIV positive and had used heroin daily for more than five years found that after being treated for malnutrition and rehabilitated from drug use, none had developed symptoms or infections associated with AIDS an average of four years after testing positive.[234]

- People who shun or stop AIDS treatment drugs after testing HIV positive and live in uncompromised good health, and people who quit AIDS drugs and remain alive and well many years after an AIDS diagnosis are not a focus of orthodox AIDS research, are rarely mentioned in mainstream AIDS literature, and are not objectively examined in government-funded AIDS studies.

- Books and articles by and about healthy HIV positives emphasize the use of nutrition and vitamin therapy and other forms of natural, holistic, and nontoxic treatments that replenish and fortify immune health.[235]

- Lymphoma, diarrhea, dementia, candidiasis, neuropathy, nausea, wasting, bone marrow destruction, and many other conditions that define or are associated with AIDS are among the effects of the prescription drugs used to treat AIDS.

- "Early intervention" and **prophylaxis** are concepts that can bring about lethal consequences. Taking AZT or other chemotherapy as antivirals, or using powerful antibiotics such as Bactrim every day for months to years, is a new and

Prophylaxis: The prevention of or protective treatment for disease.

potentially deadly practice that defies both the manufacturers' warnings and the recommended usage as outlined in the *Physician's Desk Reference* (PDR).

- T cell measures are of questionable value as an indicator of health and immune function. In fact, a decrease in T cell counts is neither necessary nor sufficient for the appearance of AIDS-defining illnesses.[236]

- A number of studies found in the biomedical literature show that low T cell counts do not correlate with compromised immunity, and that normal ranges for T cells in HIV negative persons can vary from 300 to 2,000.[237,238]

- A study of T cell measures in 2,000 HIV negative subjects demonstrated that counts of 200 and 300 are within the parameters of normal, and that people with T cells in this range did not suffer from health problems related to immune deficiency.[237] A more recent article from the medical literature questions the value of T cell counts as indicators of immune function, noting that the ability to recover from illness does not correlate with high T cells counts.[239]

- Other studies that measure T cells in HIV negative subjects reveal that even during acute illness, T cell counts are unpredictable and do not correlate with the severity of illness, or with predicted or actual mortality rates.[240]

- As noted previously, viral load tests are not able to confirm the presence of HIV and results do not correlate with illness, health, T cells levels or progression to disease.

- According to CDC treatment guidelines, acute illness (such as bacterial and pneumocystis pneumonia) and immunizations can cause elevated viral load test results for several weeks.[241]

- Contrary to popular belief, an AIDS diagnosis is not an immutable death sentence. Safe and effective treatments that address specific, individual needs make recovery from even the most serious conditions a reality.

Options for Healing and Wellness[242]

The alternatives to orthodox Western medicine mentioned here share several common features: They were established long before our current scientific approaches to explaining and dealing with wellness and illness; rather than being disease-oriented therapies, they are methods for restoring and maintaining health; and all work with respect to the body's natural ability to heal. None offer quick-fix solutions but require participation in a process in which patient and practitioner work together to articulate and achieve goals. Some methods necessitate major life changes, others may become a catalyst for new approaches to living.

Herbal Therapy

Until the beginning of modern science and chemistry, almost all medicines were herbs. Herbal remedies were first systematized in ancient Rome, Greece, Egypt and China. Herbs are natural medicines that contain a variety of biologically active ingredients and are used to successfully treat allergies, bacterial and viral infections, chronic fatigue, immune disorders, fever, cuts, burns, rashes, and reproductive problems. They can also be used as relaxants and stimulants. About 25% of conventional pharmaceuticals include synthetic forms of herbs.

Herbs are generally safer and gentler than prescription drugs, and often more effective. In many instances, they work in areas where Western medical treatments fail. Herbal remedies can be used for prevention of illness, as complementary substances with drugs, or in place of pharmaceuticals. Because certain herbs can be toxic, following the advice of a health professional or a detailed guidebook is recommended.

Herbs are used fresh or dried, can be prepared in capsules, pills, powders, concentrated liquids, extracts and teas. They can also be applied topically in creams or ointments, and used as compresses or poultices.

Nutritional Medicine

Nutritional healing is a natural method of overcoming illness and maintaining wellness without the use of toxic drugs. Nutritional medicine recognizes the body as a complex biochemical system that has specific requirements for optimal function. In addition to proteins, fats, carbohydrates, and water, there are over 40 different vitamins, minerals, fatty acids, amino acids and other components—including oxygen and sunlight—that are necessary for maintaining wellness. A deficiency in any of these essential nutrients will result in some form of ill-health ranging from a barely perceptible or subclinical problem to serious and even life-threatening disease. While single deficiencies are rare, multiple subclinical deficiencies are common among people with a typical Western diet which is characterized by an excess of processed foods that are high in fat and sugar, and lacking in whole, fresh foods that provide vital nutrients.

Nutritional medicine uses dietary changes, vitamins, minerals, herbs, and other supplements to encourage the entire body to heal itself. In this manner, the cause of disease or illness, not just the symptoms, are alleviated. Although there are general rules for proper nutrition, each person has a unique body chemistry that affects how they respond to nutrients. What works quickly and well for some may not work at all for others. In cases of serious or chronic illness, it is important to seek individualized care that can identify digestive malfunctions and toxic buildup. Also, vitamins and minerals interact in complex ways and are absorbed differently by each person.

Naturopathic Medicine

Naturopathy is a system of medicine that promotes health by stimulating and supporting the body's inherent power to heal. Although the term naturopathy was first adopted in the early 1900s, its philosophical basis dates back as far as 400 BC. A naturopathic doctor, or ND, seeks to discover and alleviate the root causes of disease rather than eliminating or suppressing symptoms, works with a patient to create conditions that enhance healing, and avoids drugs and surgery whenever possible. Since physical and psychological elements are recognized to contribute to disease, NDs generally pay considerable attention to a patient's lifestyle.

Treatments include dietary changes and nutritional therapy, herbs, vitamins and other supplements, and forms of physical exercise. Naturopaths may use a number of alternative therapies including homeopathy and traditional Oriental Medicine. The naturopathic approach emphasizes education and endeavors to provide the patient with information on what they can do independently to maintain or improve health.

Homeopathy

Founded in 1790, homeopathy comes from two words, *homeo* meaning similar, and *pathy* designating disease. Homeopathy is commonly practiced in many countries including France, India, Mexico, Russia, and England, where one in three people—including the royal family—use homeopathy as their primary form of medical care. Introduced to the US in 1825, by 1890 there were 14,000 homeopathic physicians, 22 homeopathic medical schools and 100 homeopathic hospitals nationwide. Fifty years later, regulation by and reliance on Western medicine had driven homeopathy to near extinction. But today, more than 2.5 million Americans seek homeopathic care each year.

According to the principles of homeopathy, disease represents an imbalance in the immune system, and a small stimulus can restore the balance of the body's natural defenses. Homeopathy operates on the Law of Similars, the principle that "like cures like." For example, a person suffering with diarrhea would be given a highly diluted amount of a substance that induces diarrhea, thus stimulating natural healing mechanisms. Homeopathy has proved particularly helpful in resolving chronic and transient conditions such as asthma, allergies, arthritis, colds and flu.

Rather than treating specific diseases or problems, homeopaths treat the whole person based on an assessment of all physical and emotional symptoms, and do not necessarily employ the same remedies for different people with the same problem. However, over-the-counter homeopathic combinations are safely and successfully used for fever, swelling, muscle aches, nausea, vomiting, diarrhea, food poisoning, insect bites, headaches, earaches, colds and flu, and many other problems.

Detoxification and Cleansing

The role of cleansing in recovery, wellness and immune system fortification is commonly underestimated despite the fact that most all health professionals will agree that a sick body is a toxic body. Cleansing rids the body of toxins, allowing the organs and body systems to rejuvenate themselves naturally.

Toxic acids are by-products of normal metabolic changes in cells known as cell catabolism. We also take in varying amounts of toxic materials from air, water and other environmental sources, from the herbicides, pesticides and chemical additives in food, as well as from prescription and street drugs. The body's ability to clear away the toxic materials created and assimilated each day is vital to health and immune response. Problems occur when these poisons accumulate faster than they are eliminated or when one or more of the systems designed to rid the body of toxins is underactive. Health and recovery programs that use detoxification and cleansing aid the body's natural systems that eliminate poisons, and facilitate the rebuilding of body tissues.

Colon hydrotherapy, juice fasting and diets, herbs, vitamins, minerals, and enzymes are used for detoxification and cleansing purposes. Some of these methods can be employed without professional supervision, but in the case of serious illness, it is important to regulate the amount of toxins released into the bloodstream during cleansing.

Ayurvedic Medicine

Ayurveda is a unique approach to physical health, mental clarity, and even spiritual fulfillment that began in India more than 5,000 years ago. The term Ayurveda derives from the Sanskrit roots *ayur* which means life, and *veda* meaning knowledge. The three *doshas* or body types—*vata*, *pitta* and *kapha*—are the cornerstone of Ayurvedic diagnosis and treatment. Determining a *dosha* involves gathering specific information on physical and psychological history and tendencies in order to create a detailed portrait of a type of individual.

Every person has a different mixture of *doshas*; usually one is most prominent and another is secondary. According to Ayurveda, keeping the *doshas* in balance can facilitate healing and lead to a healthier and longer life. Specific health problems may also be alleviated through Ayurvedic medicine.

Ayuverdic practitioners generally prescribe a variety of foods, herbs, exercises, breathing techniques, massages and *dosha*-specific diets with the goal of detoxifying and balancing the system.

Acupuncture and Chinese Herbology

A major component of Oriental Medicine, acupuncture works by altering the internal flow of vital life energy or *chi*. This life energy moves along established pathways or meridians in the body that relate to the organs and the tendo-muscular system. When the balance of *chi* is disturbed due to physical or emotional trauma, poor diet, pharmaceuticals, stress, genetic or environmental factors, pain or illness result. Inserting hair-thin needles at specific meridian points restores the balance of *chi* by calming, strengthening or removing a blockage of the flow. An average acupuncture treatment involves five to 15 needles in a procedure that usually causes little discomfort. In addition to, or sometimes instead of inserting needles, an acupuncturist may use a treatment called moxibustion in which heat is applied directly above acupuncture points.

Acupuncture is generally used in conjunction with Chinese Herbology. Both are safe medical procedures that are known for their efficacy and lack of adverse side effects. Doctors of Oriental Medicine, or OMDs, prescribe herbal combinations according to a complex system of diagnosis. These herbal formulas are intended to help the body correct imbalances of energy while stimulating the natural healing process. A number of clinical and laboratory studies have generated scientific evidence that herbs can effectively treat many diseases. Herb formulas may be prepared in pills, capsules, granules, tinctures or teas, and are an important part of the traditional system of Oriental Medicine.

Imagery

The concept that imagination has the ability to cure illness is not new. Ancient Greeks and Egyptians believed that images release spirits in the brain that stimulate various organs and functions, and that a mental picture of disease is enough to cause its symptoms. In the 1600s, imagery was thought to wield such power that it could even affect embryos in pregnant women. One hundred years later, doctors and healers changed their minds and agreed with French philosopher René Descartes who asserted that the mind and body were separate and had no influence on each other.

Imagery came back into practice in the 1970s as a method for helping cancer patients. In one landmark study, cancer patients who used imagery in conjunction with standard medical care lived twice as long as those receiving medical care alone.

Several studies suggest that imagery can boost immune response. Imagery has been used to increase activity of natural killer cells that recognize and destroy virus-infected cells, other microbes, and tumor cells. Other studies have shown that imagery can lower blood pressure, slow heart rate, alleviate insomnia, relieve stress and anxiety, treat phobias and obesity, and help regulate menstrual cycles. PET scans (positron-emission-tomography tests that highlight areas of brain activity) have demonstrated that the brain can react the same way to an imagined sensation as a real one.

Recommended Reading for Healing and Wellness

Alternative Medicine: The Definitive Guide
The Burton Goldberg Group
Future Medicine Publishing, Inc.

New Choices in Natural Healing
Bill Gottlieb, Editor
Rodale Press, Inc.

The Illustrated Encyclopedia of Healing Remedies
Norman Shealy, MD, PhD
Element Books Limited

Complete Encyclopedia of Natural Healing
Gary Null, PhD
Kensington Books

The Complete Illustrated Guide to Nutritional Healing
Denise Mortimore
Element Press

Prescription for Nutritional Healing
James Balch, MD
Avery Publishing Group

The Food Pharmacy
Jean Carper
Bantam Books

Homeopathic Medicine at Home
Maesimund Panos, MD
JP Tarcher

Asian Health Secrets: The Complete Guide to Asian Herbal Medicine
Letha Hadady, DAc
Three Rivers Press

You Don't Have to Die Sick: The Immune Booster Resource Guide
Bob L. Owen, PhD, DSc
HealthHope Publishing House

Beyond Antibiotics: 50 Ways to Boost Immunity and Avoid Antibiotics
Dr. Michael Schmidt
North Atlantic Books

How to Survive Medical Treatment: A Holistic Guide to Avoiding Risks and Side Effects of Conventional Medicine
Dr. Stephen Fulder, MD
CW Daniel

Prescription Alternatives
Earl Mindell, RPh, PhD
Keats Publishing

Earl Mindell's Vitamin Bible for the 21st Century
Earl Mindell, RPh, PhD
Warner Books

Your Liver...Your Lifeline: Detoxification and Rejuvenation for the Whole Body
Jack Tips, PhD
Apple-A-Day Press

Tissue Cleansing Through Bowel Management
Bernard Jensen, PhD, DC
Bernard Jensen International

Cleanse and Purify Thyself
Richard Anderson, ND, NMD
Triumph

Miracles Do Happen: A Physician's Experience with Alternative Medicine
Norman Shealy, MD, PhD
Element Books Limited

Quantum Healing: Exploring the Frontiers of Mind/Body Medicine
Deepak Chopra, MD
Bantam Books

Why People Don't Heal and How They Can
Caroline Myss, PhD
Three Rivers Press

How to Raise a Healthy Child...In Spite of Your Doctor
Robert Mendelsohn, MD
Ballantine Books

What You Can Do to End AIDS

Solutions to AIDS will only come about through unbiased examination of facts and open, honest dialogue. You can help create the changes needed to end the AIDS crisis now.

Learn more: Check out the books from our recommended reading list, visit the various web sites, and subscribe to the publications described on page 78.

Spread the word: Use the form on page 127 to order additional copies of this book to share with concerned friends, healthcare professionals, educators, student groups, the media, policy makers and government officials. Donate copies to your local public library, your school, your church or other community groups. Ask local health and book stores to carry our book. For information on quantity or commercial orders or to locate a distributor near you, contact us toll-free at (877) 92-ALIVE.

Link to our website: Visit us at *www.aliveandwell.org* and sign our international petition for a reappraisal of AIDS.

Share your story: If this book has changed your views on HIV and AIDS, let us know. If you are HIV positive, healthy and live without AIDS treatment drugs, send us your story. Help us provide others with realistic hope and vital information that major media and AIDS groups ignore.

Invite us to share our story: The author and noted members of The American Foundation for AIDS Alternative's scientific advisory board are available for public events. Call us for more information.

Support our work: Send a tax-deductible donation. The American Foundation for AIDS Alternatives is one of the only AIDS organizations that does not solicit or accept funding from the pharmaceutical industry, the US government or any entity that limits the questions we may ask or the answers we may receive about HIV, AIDS and health.

The American Foundation for AIDS Alternatives works locally by sponsoring free monthly community events and classes, and works globally by sharing our ideas, experience, resources and funds with other AIDS reappraisal groups around the country, and throughout the world. We also sponsor scientific and medical research studies that examine alternative approaches to resolving AIDS.

Sources for Further Information

Books

The HIV Myth
Jad Adams
St. Martin's Press

Sex at Risk
Stuart Brody
Transaction Publishers

Black Lies, White Lies
Tony Brown
William Morrow and Company

The AIDS Mirage
Hiram Caton, PhD
www.users.bigpond.com/smartboard/aids

Infectious AIDS: Have We Been Misled?
Peter Duesberg, PhD
North Atlantic Books

Inventing the AIDS Virus
Peter Duesberg, PhD
Regnery Publishing

The Myth of Heterosexual AIDS
Michael Fumento
Basic Books

AIDS: The Failure of Contemporary Science
Neville Hodgkinson
Fourth Estate Press

Challenges
Serge Lange, PhD
Springer

The AIDS Cult
John Lauritsen and Ian Young
Askelpios/Pagan Press

The AIDS War
John Lauritsen
Askelpios/Pagan Press

Prescription for Profits
Linda Marsa
Scribner

AIDS Inc.: Scandal of the Century
Jon Rappoport
Human Energy Press

Positively False
Joan Shenton
IB Tauris

Websites

AIDS Coalition To Unleash Power: ACT UP San Francisco
www.actupsf.com

AIDS Authority
www.aidsauthority.org/main.html

Alive & Well AIDS Alternatives
www.aliveandwell.org

Continuum
www.continuum.org.uk

HEAL
www.healaids.com

Impression Magazine
www.ironminds.com/impression/index.shtml

International Coalition for Medical Justice (ICMJ)
www.icmj.org

Mothering Magazine
www.mothering.com

New African Magazine
www.africasia.com/icpubs/na/naconts.htm

Rethinking AIDS
www.rethinkingaids.com

Sumeria: The Immune System
www.thuntek.net/sumeria/aids.html

Virus Myth
www.virusmyth.com

Organizations

ACT UP Hollywood

8965 Santa Monica Blvd., PMB #157 • West Hollywood, CA 90069
Tel: (323) 692-7766 • Email: actuphollywood@yahoo.com

ACT UP San Francisco

1884 Market Street • San Francisco, CA 94102
Tel: (415) 864-6686 • Fax: (415) 864-6687 • Email: actupsf@aol.com

ACT UP is determined to end AIDS through militant direct action. We confront complacency, conflict of interest and corruption in the AIDS industry. We protest homophobia, racism, sexism and poverty as the causes of ill health. ACT UP does not accept contributions from pharmaceutical companies or the government.

Alberta Reappraising AIDS Society

David Crowe, President
Box 61037 • Kensington Postal Outlet • Calgary, Alberta T2N 4S6, Canada
Tel: (403) 220-0129 • Email: 71574,3157@compuserve.com

Alberta Reappraising AIDS Society uses scientific evidence to challenge the myth that HIV is the cause of AIDS, and specifically to question the use of toxic compounds to fight AIDS. Goals are accomplished through education, lobbying and, if necessary, legal action in the province of Alberta, Canada.

Alive & Well AIDS Alternatives

Christine Maggiore, Director
11684 Ventura Boulevard • Studio City, CA 91604
Toll-Free: (877) 92-ALIVE • Fax: (818) 780-7093
Email: christine@aliveandwell.org

Alive & Well questions the HIV=AIDS=Death paradigm based on a growing body of scientific, medical, and epidemiological data, and promotes awareness of life-affirming facts to HIV positive diagnosed persons and concerned citizens worldwide. In addition to sponsoring scientific and medical studies, Alive & Well offers a yearly calendar of free community events, produces books, videos, and other materials that present alternative views of AIDS, and shares resources with Alive & Well affiliates and other organizations around the world that support informed choices for people affected by HIV and AIDS.

The Group for the Scientific Reappraisal of the HIV/AIDS Hypothesis

Dr. David Rasnick, President
7514 Girard Avenue #1-331 • La Jolla, CA 92037
Toll-Free: (877) 256-6406 • Fax: (619)272-1621 • Email: editor@rethinkingaids.com

The Group for the Scientific Reappraisal of the HIV/AIDS Hypothesis comprises medical scientists, physicians, other professionals and concerned people who conclude that HIV might not explain AIDS and that everyone should think and speak freely on this topic without fear of professional, social, or academic reprisals. The Group publishes the monthly newsletter *Rethinking AIDS*.

HEAL (Health Education AIDS Liaison)

Michael Ellner, President, Founding HEAL Chapter
PO Box 1103 • Old Chelsea Station • New York, NY 10113
Tel: (212) 873-0780 • Fax: (212) 873-0891 • Email: revdocnyc@aol.com

Ron Piazza, National Contact for Independent Chapters, USA
Toll-Free: (800) 738-3642 • Email: heal@seanet.com

HEAL, Independent Chapters, Canada

Carl Strygg, Robert Johnston, Co-founders
993 Queen Street East • Toronto, Ontario M4M1K2, Canada
Tel: (416) 406-HEAL • Fax: (416) 778-7381 • Email: endaids@hotmail.com

HEAL provides information needed to make truly informed decisions about HIV testing and treatments. Some HEAL chapters offer natural and nontoxic alternatives to these treatments. Others offer insight into the wider social context for the complex of noninfectious health risks that cause AIDS. Write or call for more information, and a complete list of independent HEAL chapters and/or affiliates in the US, Canada and other parts of the world.

International Coalition for Medical Justice (ICMJ)

Deane Collie, Executive Director • Robert Beard, Chief Counsel
302 East Davis Street, Suite 221 • Culpepper, VA 22701
Tel: (540) 829-9350 • Fax: (540) 829-9009 • Email: ICMJ@biosys.net

ICMJ promotes and encourages ethical and responsible scientific research methods and advocates true informed consent for medical treatment methods. ICMJ provides grant funding for research and education, as well as legal defense and legal defense funding.

Mothers Opposing Mandatory Medicine

11684 Ventura Boulevard • Studio City, CA 91604
Toll-Free: (877) 804-4MOM • Fax: (818) 780-7093
Email: momm@aliveandwell.org

MOMM provides critical education and peer support to expectant and current mothers faced with choices regarding HIV testing and pharmaceutical HIV and AIDS treatments, and offers information on healthy childbirth, breastfeeding, and living in wellness.

The National Vaccine Information Center

512 West Maple Avenue, Suite 206 • Vienna, VA 22180
Tel: (703) 938-0342 • Fax: (703) 938-5768

The National Vaccine Information Center (NVIC), founded in 1982 by parents of vaccine injured children, is a nonprofit, educational organization dedicated to preventing vaccine injuries and deaths through public education and defending the right of all citizens to informed consent to vaccination. NVIC takes the position that scientific evidence to date is not sufficient to prove HIV causes AIDS and that if an HIV vaccine is made available to the public in the future, no citizen should be required to use it without their voluntary, informed consent. NVIC maintains that the ethical principle of informed consent, which is applied to all other medical procedures carrying a risk of injury or death, must be applied to all vaccinations, including a future AIDS vaccine.

Students Reappraising AIDS

Kai Thorup, Director
2880 SW 75th Way #2205 • Davie, FL 33314
Toll-Free: (877) 411-AIDS • Florida: (954) 382-9995 • Email: kai@thorup.com

Students Reappraising AIDS encourages students to raise questions that challenge the HIV=AIDS=Death paradigm in their classrooms, among their fellow students and on their campuses by providing a forum for scientists, physicians, journalists and activists to present factual information that exposes the myth that HIV causes AIDS.

Publications

Rethinking AIDS

7514 Girard Avenue #1-331 • La Jolla, CA 92037
Toll-Free: (877) 256-6406 • Fax: (619) 272-1621
Email: editor@rethinkingaids.com

Rethinking AIDS is the monthly publication of The Group for the Scientific Reappraisal of the HIV/AIDS Hypothesis. Every issue offers easily understandable and highly informative insights into the facts behind current AIDS news. An excellent guide to understanding the latest claims, numbers, and studies from the AIDS establishment. Annual subscriptions are available for a tax deductible $25 donation for US addresses ($35 international). US residents are invited to call toll-free to request a complimentary sample issue.

Continuum

4A Hollybush Place • London E2 9QX • England, UK
Tel: 440-171-613-3909 • Fax: 440-171-613-312
Email: continu@dircon.co.uk • Website: www.continuum.org.uk

A full-size magazine published bimonthly in England. Covers AIDS news and events from around the globe and features extensive articles on alternatives to pharmaceutical therapies and standard AIDS-think. Produced by an international nonprofit group of HIV positives, a free trial copy is available on request. Credit cards accepted.

Subscription rates in US dollars (individual/organization)

	UK	European Union	Elsewhere
6 issues	$40 / $60	$49 / $73	$52 / $78
12 issues	$75 / $105	$90 / $132	$96 / $141
18 issues	$112 / $150	$135 / $190	$144 / $204

Understanding AIDS Speak: A Guide to Language in the Age of HIV

AIDS: Popularly referred to as a disease, AIDS is actually a new name for 29 previously known and relatively common health conditions when these conditions appear in someone who has tested HIV positive. For example, a person who tests HIV positive and has herpes is classified as having AIDS, while a person with herpes who tests HIV negative has herpes, not AIDS. All 29 health conditions categorized as AIDS occur in people who test HIV negative, and none are exclusive to those who test HIV positive. "AIDS" is not a disease, just as "hardware" is not a tool— both are categories that are used to group certain items.

AIDS Education/AIDS Awareness: Presentation of popular beliefs, unsubstantiated claims and unfounded projections regarding HIV and AIDS which excludes all or most of the factual information contained in this book.

AIDS Epidemic: An epidemic is generally defined as an outbreak of a contagious disease that spreads rapidly, grows quickly and is widely prevalent. Since 1981, AIDS has remained almost exclusively confined to the original risk groups, has not spread rapidly among risk group members, and is not widely prevalent anywhere in the world. For example, 99.5% of people living on the African continent, an area often described as being devastated by AIDS, do not have AIDS.

AIDS Infected: A misleading, incongruous phrase popularized by the media to describe people with a positive result on a nonspecific test for antibodies thought to be associated with HIV. There is no such thing as an "AIDS infection."

AIDS-Related: Any troublesome health condition that is not included in the official definition of AIDS, yet is attributed to AIDS, but only in a person who has tested HIV positive. For example, Arthur Ashe is reported to have died of "AIDS-related pneumonia," a pneumonia that is not an AIDS-defining illness.[243] Most AIDS-related conditions are caused by AIDS treatments, as in AIDS-related anemia, and are treated with other AIDS drugs. Some, like AIDS-related gum disease, or gingivitis, are problems commonly found in the general population.

AIDS Test: What is popularly known as an "AIDS test" is actually a test for antibodies generated to act against HIV yet HIV tests are not able to specifically identify antibodies to HIV. Viral antibodies alone cannot cause and do not predict illness. HIV antibody tests are nonspecific, highly cross-reactive and do not detect HIV (actual virus). There is no test to diagnose AIDS.

AIDS Vaccine Program: A multi-billion dollar research effort to create a vaccine against AIDS that will cause a person to produce antibodies to HIV. All vaccines work by artificially stimulating production of antibodies which then serve as protection from a specific disease. Researchers say that the antibodies to HIV elicited by a vaccine will protect people from AIDS even though naturally occurring HIV antibodies are considered an indicator of current or impending illness. As participants in AIDS vaccine trials become HIV positive after vaccination, researchers have discovered that there is no way of distinguishing the HIV antibodies induced by the vaccine from naturally occurring HIV antibodies. A recent article in the journal *Lancet* reported on this dilemma: Researchers attempting to determine who was HIV positive due to vaccination found that viral load tests commonly used by AIDS doctors to diagnose HIV infection were "unsuitable for diagnostic screening" when positive samples from one lab were found to be negative at another.[244] The problem of distinguishing people who have been immunized against HIV from those with naturally acquired HIV antibodies is described in the report as "increasingly complicated, raising critical questions for the conduct of all HIV vaccine trials."

AIDS Virus: A popular name for HIV, a retrovirus with no cell-killing mechanisms that has not been found in the fresh, uncultured plasma of AIDS patients or in persons diagnosed as HIV positive.

Antivirals/Antiretrovirals: Chemotherapy drug compounds designed to terminate forming DNA chains. None of the many drugs commonly referred to as antivirals or antiretrovirals possess any direct or specific mechanisms for targeting virus. Actual antiviral drugs do not exist, as medical science has never produced a drug that can cure a viral infection.

At Risk: According to AIDS organizations, the media and government advertising campaigns, everyone is at risk for AIDS although for nearly two decades, over 90% of American AIDS cases are confined to groups with well-known risk factors not shared by the general American population. As early as 1987, the CDC acknowledged that "most people are at zilcho or very low risk" and that the chance of acquiring HIV from a one-time unprotected heterosexual encounter with someone not in a high risk group is one in seven million, which is smaller than the risk of ever being struck by lightning.[245] As reported in *The Wall Street Journal*, government health officials decided in 1988 to portray AIDS as an "equal opportunity scourge" because market research indicated that such a claim would "mobilize support for public funding" and "generate compassion for victims."

Chronic and Manageable: The new goal of conventional AIDS science, as in "the new drugs could make AIDS a chronic and manageable condition."

Compassionate Use/Expanded Access: Making experimental, unproven, or previously banned drugs available for use outside of experimental trials. For example, thalidomide, a drug banned in the 1960s for causing severe birth defects was recently released for compassionate use as a treatment for AIDS wasting, a condition known to be caused by other AIDS drugs.

Compliance: Strictly adhering to an intricate and complex program of AIDS drugs as if one's life depended on it.

Early Intervention: Pharmaceutical treatment of illness before illness occurs, also known as prophylaxis. Presumption of illness and prediction of future illness in persons who test HIV positive are based on highly biased statistical data and surrogate markers rather than on individual clinical health status. Early intervention often produces the dire health consequences it is used to prevent. Synonymous with "aggressive treatment," "hitting early and hard" and "being smart about HIV."

Early Intervention Specialists/Treatment Advisors/Treatment Advocates: Functionaries of AIDS organizations who promote pharmaceuticals, often to the exclusion of alternative treatments and approaches to living. Many AIDS organizations do not allow people serving in this capacity to mention information on healthful living without drug intervention.

Failing Drug Therapy: Describes a person who is unable to tolerate the side effects of AIDS drugs, or for whom the drugs produce no beneficial results; as in "John failed Crixivan." According to this cruel paradigm, drugs do not fail, people do.

Fast-Tracking/Fast-Track Approval: Releasing pharmaceutical treatments for general and lifelong use before long-term results are known and before safety and efficacy have been established. Many adverse effects of protease inhibitors—sexual dysfunction, diabetes, physical deformities, liver failure, and death—were discovered only after fast-track release. Fast-tracking is regarded as one of the major accomplishments of AIDS activism.

Fatal: Describes conditions, circumstances or events that have produced death or are destined inevitably to cause death.[246] According to the World Health Organization, 95% of people worldwide described as "having HIV" actually live in health despite promotions of HIV as a 100% fatal virus.[247]

Fighting AIDS: Funding AIDS.

Full-Blown AIDS: Testing HIV positive and meeting the criteria for an AIDS diagnosis by having any official AIDS-defining condition ranging from a simple yeast infection to terminal cancer, as in "Mary has full-blown AIDS." Since January of 1993, a diagnosis of full-blown AIDS does not require that a person have any illness.

HIV Positive: Used to describe someone who has tested positive for antibodies presumed to have been produced in response to HIV. A diagnosis of HIV positive does not refer to actual infection with HIV and may vary depending on where one lives. Popularly considered synonymous with a death sentence. People who test positive may be charged with felony offenses for having sexual relations, and may lose custody of their children for their healthcare choices.

In Denial: Anyone who questions the HIV hypothesis. Most often applied to HIV positives who refuse pharmaceutical treatment and choose to live.

Infected: See HIV Positive.

Informed Choices: What people who test HIV positive are said to make after being provided with information through AIDS organizations and drug company-sponsored seminars that exclude the facts found in this book.

Inhumane/Unethical: The use of unmedicated placebo controls in studies that test proposed AIDS treatment drugs. Until recently, the placebo control was regarded as a necessary procedure that provided a scientific basis for evaluation of drug treatments and enabled more accurate assessments of drug efficacy.

Long-Term Survivor: A person who tests HIV positive and remains alive for more than three to five years. Differs from a long-term non-progressor in that a long-term survivor need only be alive and not necessarily in good health. Many long-term survivors live with drug side effects such as chronic diarrhea and nausea, wasting, anemia or neuropathy.

Mutation: A popular notion used to explain why the effects of AIDS drugs are nonexistent or short-lived. This idea presumes that HIV develops into mutant strains that resist drug therapy although there is no scientific evidence to substantiate such a notion, and evidence for drug-resistant HIV viruses has not been published in the medical literature.

99% Accuracy: Alleged accuracy of HIV antibody tests which do not specifically identify antibodies to HIV, that cross-react with many non-HIV antibodies, that are not standardized and have not been verified against virus isolation in people who test positive.

Non-Progressors: People who test HIV positive, take no AIDS treatments and enjoy good health. Many scientists hypothesize that such people are infected with a less virulent strain of HIV, or imagine that they possess a unique gene that protects them from developing AIDS. Scientists have speculated that African-Americans do not possess this unidentified gene.[248] A portion of the multi-billion dollar AIDS research effort is directed to a search for the presumed gene.

Otherwise Healthy: Most commonly used to describe chronic users of recreational and pharmaceutical drugs, people chronically exposed to numerous infectious microbes, the malnourished, hemophiliacs and transfusion recipients, and impoverished residents of developing nations who develop symptoms of immune deficiency diseases, but only if they also test HIV positive. Also used to describe people who test HIV positive and have no health problems. See *Non-Progressors*.

Resistance: What AIDS patients are said to develop when AIDS drugs fail to produce benefits or when temporary effects cease entirely. Benefits of drug treatments generally have no relation to actual health and are instead determined by certain blood test results known as surrogate markers. See *Mutation*.

Side Effects: The direct unwanted or unintended results of treatment with pharmaceuticals or other substances.

Surrogate Markers: In AIDS, the laboratory tests that measure T cells or purport to quantify "viral load." Surrogate markers have replaced actual health as measures of actual health. The efficacy of AIDS drugs is determined by changes in surrogate markers that do not correlate with actual health.

Viral Load: A hypothetical notion that HIV reproduces as many as one billion times daily, and that the quantities of HIV produced every day kill off the enormous number of T cells produced every day, causing the immune destruction associated with AIDS. The concept of viral load does not explain how HIV actually kills T cells, why the billions of "virus" it finds are not detectable by any means normally used to detect virus, or why significant quantities of HIV cannot be isolated from the fresh, uncultured plasma of people who test HIV positive or who have illnesses defined as AIDS.

Viral Load Test: The name given to a laboratory test which does not measure or identify HIV (actual virus) and is prohibited for use by the FDA for confirming the presence of HIV or diagnosing viral infection. This test is commonly used to diagnose HIV infection and serves as a basis for prescribing medication that includes toxic, experimental chemicals to symptomless HIV positives, pregnant women, infants and children.

Wasting Syndrome: An AIDS condition that is characterized by atrophy of body mass and involuntary weight loss. Almost every AIDS drug from Bactrim to protease inhibitors causes chronic diarrhea resulting in weight loss; AZT and other nucleoside analogs known as antivirals are acknowledged to cause deterioration of muscle mass. Many persons with an HIV positive diagnosis take combinations of such drugs on a regular, ongoing basis.

References

1. In the United States, AIDS = 28 old illnesses and one non-illness:

   1983 original AIDS definition (12 illnesses): Pneumocystis carinii pneumonia, Kaposi's sarcoma, toxoplasmosis, strongyloidosis, aspergillosis, cryptococcosis, candidiasis, cryptosporidiosis, cytomegalovirus, herpes simplex, progressive multifocal leukoencephalopathy, lymphoma of the brain

   1985 revised definition (seven more old illnesses added): Mycobacterium avium complex, histoplasmosis, isosporiasis, Burkitt's lymphoma, immunoblastic lymphoma, candidiasis of the bronchi, trachea and lungs, and a positive HIV antibody test.

   1987 revised definition (six additional illnesses): Encephalopathy, Mycobacterium tuberculosis, wasting syndrome, coccidioidomycosis, cytomegalovirus retinitis, Salmonella septicemia. HIV antibody test no longer required.

   1993 revised definition (three more illnesses plus one surrogate marker): Recurrent bacterial pneumonia, invasive cervical cancer, pulmonary tuberculosis, T Cell count of <200 or <14% of total lymphocytes (non-illness).

   Source: Duesberg P, Yiamouyannis J, 1995 *AIDS: The Good News Is HIV Doesn't Cause It* Health Action Press
2. US Centers for Disease Control 1994 *HIV/AIDS Surveillance Report* Year-end edition 1993
3. Navarro M *AIDS Definition Widened to Include Blood Cell Count* August 8 1993 New York Times; Altman L *AIDS Cases Increase Among Heterosexuals* March 11 1994 New York Times
4. US Centers for Disease Control *HIV/AIDS Surveillance Report* Year-end editions 1998, 1997, 1996, 1995, 1994, 1993
5. US Centers for Disease Control 1998 *HIV/AIDS Surveillance Report* Year-end edition 1997 Table 11 p17
6. US Centers for Disease Control 1999 *HIV/AIDS Surveillance Report* Year-end edition 1998 p43
7. Duesberg P 1993 *The HIV Gap in National Statistics* Bio/Technology 11:955-6
8. Laboratory Centre for Disease Control, Health Canada, 1998 *HIV and AIDS in Canada: Surveillance Report to December 31, 1997*; US Centers for Disease Control 1999 *HIV/AIDS Surveillance Report* Year-end 1998
9. US Centers for Disease Control 1998 *HIV/AIDS Surveillance Report* Year-end edition 1997 Figure 6 p25; US Centers for Disease Control 1999 *HIV/AIDS Surveillance Report* Year-end edition 1998
10. World Health Organization 1985 Bangui definition for AIDS in Africa (current use confirmed by WHO April 1999); WHO case definitions for AIDS surveillance in adults and adolescents, *Weekly Epidemiological Record* September 1994; 69:273–80 (current use confirmed by WHO April 1999)
11. Duesberg P 1996 *Inventing the AIDS Virus* Regnery Press, Washington DC p141–145
12. Duesberg P 1996 *Inventing the AIDS Virus* Regnery Press, Washington DC p54–58
13. Carins J 1978 *Cancer: Science and Society* WH Freeman and Company, San Francisco
14. Duesberg P, Rasnick D 1998 *The AIDS Dilemma: Drug Diseases Blamed on a Passenger Virus* Genetica 104:85-132; Mullis K 1998 *Dancing Naked in the Mindfield* Pantheon Books, New York p171–190; Shenton J 1998 *Positively False* St Martin's Press, New York p6–17
15. Mullis K 1988 *Dancing Naked in the Mindfield* Pantheon Books, New York p 178; Duesberg P 1996 *Inventing the AIDS Virus* Regnery Press, Washington DC p 89–96
16. Altman L New York Times, April 23 1984
17. Altman L *Researchers Believe AIDS Virus is Found* New York Times, April 24 1984 (Dr. James Curran, head of the CDC's AIDS investigating team, calls discovery "the virus that causes AIDS")
18. Gallo found HIV in only 26 of 63 AIDS patients (41%) Source: Gallo R May 4 1984 Science Volume 224 p502
19. In 1983, Montagnier sent Gallo "retrovirus particles" (LAV) taken from the lymph node of a male homosexual without AIDS. Source: Science May 20 1983, Vol 220; the virus Gallo claimed to have discovered in 1984 was found to actually be Montagnier's LAV. Source: New Scientist, February 12 1987
20. Dingell J *Misconduct in Medical Research*, New England Journal of Medicine 1993 328:1610–1615; *Co-Discoverer of HIV Loses Bid to Regain Job* AIDS Policy and Law May 14 1999 Vol 14 No 9; Crewdson J *In Gallo Case, Truth Termed a Casualty: Science Subverted in AIDS* Research Chicago Tribune, January 1 1995
21. Baffour A *Are 26 Million Africans Dying of AIDS?* December 1998 New African Magazine p34–42
22. Duesberg P *Inventing the AIDS Virus* Regnery Press, Washington DC; Root-Bernstein R 1993 *Rethinking AIDS* The Free Press, New York
23. Cordes R, et al 1995 *Pitfalls in HIV Testing* Postgraduate Medicine 98:177; Langedijk J, et al 1992 *Identification of Cross-reaction Epitopes Recognized by HIV-1 False-positive Sera* AIDS 6:1547–1548; Strandstrom H, et al 1990 *Studies with Canine Sera that Contain Antibodies which Recognize HIV Structural Proteins* Cancer Research, September 1:50(17 Suppl):56285–56305; Germanson T 1989 *Screening for HIV: Can We Afford the Confusion of the False Positive Rate?* Journal of Clinical Epidemiology 42:1235; Weiss R, et al 1988 *HIV Testing is the Answer–What's the Question?* New England Journal of Medicine 319:1010–1012; Burke, et al 1988 *Measurement of the False Positive Rate in a Screening Program for HIV Infections* New England Journal of Medicine 319(15):961–964; US News and World Report, November 23 1987 p22c; Jackson G, et al 1988 *Passive Immunoneutralisation of Human Immunodeficiency Virus in Patients with Advanced AIDS* Lancet, September 17:647
24. Papadopulos-Eleopulos E, et al 1993 *Is a Positive Western Blot Proof of HIV Infection?* Bio/Technology Journal Vol 11 p696–707
25. Papadopulos-Eleopulos E, et al 1993 *Has Gallo Proven the Role of HIV in AIDS?* Emergency Medicine 5:113–123
26. Papadopulos-Eleopulous E, et al 1993 *Is a Positive Western Blot Proof of HIV Infection?* Bio/Technology Vol. 11
27. Strandstrom H, et al 1990 *Studies with Canine Sera which Recognise HIV Structural Proteins, Cancer Research* 50:5628s–5630s. Source: *Testing, Testing, 1,2,3...* Turner V 1996 Contiuum Vol 3:5 p8–11
28. Papadopolus-Eleopulos E, et al 1993 *Is a Positive Western Blot Proof of HIV Infection?* Bio/Technology Journal Vol 11 p696–701; Quantum Clinical

Laboratory, Los Angeles, CA: HIV antibody test results for Christine Maggiore April 9 1992 HIV reactive, WB positive positive; March 27 1993 HIV reactive, WB indeterminate; September 1 1993 HIV non-reactive

29. Abbott Laboratory's ELISA HIV antibody test kit pamphlet
30. Continuum Vol 3:4 with thanks to Val Turner, Royal Perth Hospital, Australia; Bio/Technology June 1993 11:696–707
31. Roche Amplicor PCR Diagnostics HIV-1 Monitor test kit pamphlet
32. Johnson C 1997 *Factors Known to Cause False-Positive HIV Antibody Test Results* Continuum Vol 4:3 p5

Chart References:

1c. Agbalika F, Ferchal F, et al 1992 *False-Positive Antigens Related to Emergence of a 25-30 kD Protein Detected in Organ Recipients*, AIDS 6:959-962

2c. Andrade V, Avelleira J, et al 1991 *Leprosy as a Cause of False-Positive Results in Serological Assays for the Detection of Antibodies to HIV-1* Intl J Leprosy 59:125

3c. Arnold N, Slade R, et al 1994 *Donor Follow Up of Influenza Vaccine-Related Multiple Viral Enzyme Immunoassay Reactivity* Vox Sanguinis 67:191

4c. Ascher D, Roberts C 1993 *Determination of the Etiology of Seroreversals in HIV Testing by Antibody Fingerprinting* AIDS 6:241

5c. Barbacid M, Bolgnesi D, et al 1980 *Humans Have Antibodies Capable of Recognizing Oncoviral Glycoproteins* Proceeding of The National Academy of Sciences 77:1617–1621

6c. Biggar R, Melbye M, et al 1985 *ELISA HTLV Retrovirus Antibody Reactivity Associated with Malaria and Immune Complexes in Healthy Africans* Lancet ii:520–543

7c. Blanton M, Balakrishnan K, et al 1987 *HLA Antibodies in Blood Donors with Reactive Screening Tests for Antibody to the Immunodeficiency Virus* Transfusion 27(1):118

8c. Blomberg J, Vincic E, et al 1990 *Identification of Regions of HIV-1 p24 Reactive with Sera which Give "Indeterminate" Results in Electrophoretic Immunoblots with the Help of Long Synthetic Peptides* AIDS Res Hum Retro 6:1363

9c. Burkhardt U, Mertens T, et al 1987 *Comparison of Two Commercially Available Anti-HIV ELISA's* J Med Vir 23:217

10c. Bylund D, Ziegner U, et al 1992 *Review of Testing for Human Immunodeficiency Virus* Clin Lab Med 12:305–333

11c. Challakere K, Rapaport M 1993 *False-Positive Human Immunodeficiency Virus Type 1 ELISA Results in Low-Risk Subjects* West J Med 159(2):214-215

12c. Charmot G, Simon F 1990 *HIV Infection and Malaria* Revue du practicien 40:2141

13c. Cordes R, Ryan M 1995 *Pitfalls in HIV Testing* Postgraduate Medicine 98:177

14c. Dock N, Lamberson H, et al 1988 *Evaluation of Atypical Human Immunodeficiency Virus Immunoblot Reactivity in Blood Donors* Transfusion 28:142

15c. Esteva M, Blasini A, et al 1992 *False Positive Results for Antibody to HIV in Two Men with Systemic Lupus Erythematosus* Ann Rheum Dis 51:1071–1073

16c. Fassbinder W, Kuhni P, et al 1986 *Prevalence of Antibodies Against LAV/HTLV-III [HIV] in Patients with Terminal Renal Insufficiency* Deutsche Medizinische Wochenschrift 111:1087

17c. Fleming D, Cochi S, et al 1987 *Acquired Immunodeficiency Syndrome in Low-Incidence Areas* JAMA 258(6):785

18c. Gill M, Rachlis A, et al 1991 *Five Cases of Erroneously Diagnosed HIV Infection* Can Med Asso J 145(12):1593

19c. Healey D, Bolton W 1993 *Apparent HIV-1 Glycoprotein Reactivity on Western Blot in Uninfected Blood Donors* AIDS 7:655–658

20c. Hisa J 1993 *False-Positive ELISA for Human Immunodeficiency Virus after Influenza Vaccination* JID 167:989

21c. Isaacman S 1989 *Positive HIV Antibody Test Results after Treatment with Hepatitis B Immune Globulin* JAMA 262:209

23c. Jindal R, Solomon M, et al 1993 *False Positive Tests for HIV in a Woman with Lupus and Renal Failure* NEJM 328:1281–1282

24c. Jungkind D, DiRenzo S, et al 1986 *Effect of Using Heat-Inactivated Serum with the Abbott Human T-cell Lymphotropic Virus Type III [HIV] Antibody Test* J Clin Micro 23:381

25c. Kashala O, Marlink R, et al 1994 *Infection with Human Immunodeficiency Virus Type 1 (HIV-1) and Human T-cell Lymphotropic Viruses among Leprosy Patients and Contacts* J Infect Dis 169:296–304

26c. Lai-Goldman M, McBride J, et al 1987 *Presence of HTLV-III [HIV] Antibodies in Immune Serum Globulin Preparations* Am J Clin Path 87:635

27c. Langedijk J, Vos W, et al 1992 *Identification of Cross-Reactive Epitopes Recognized by HIV-1 False-Positive Sera* AIDS 6:1547–1548

28c. Lee D, Eby W, et al 1992 *HIV False Positivity after Hepatitis B Vaccination* Lancet 339:1060

29c. Leo-Amador G, Ramirez-Rodriguez J, et al 1990 *Antibodies Against Human Immunodeficiency Virus in Generalized Lupus Erythematosus* Salud Publica de Mexico 32:15

30c. Mackenzie W, Davis J, et al 1992 *Multiple False-Positive Serologic Tests for HIV, HTLV-1 and Hepatitis C Following Influenza Vaccination, 1991* JAMA 268:1015–1017

31c. Boffey P *US to Test for AIDS in 30 Cities* New York Times December 3 1987 p31c; Mathe G 1992 *Is the AIDS Virus Responsible for the Disease?* Biomed & Pharmacother 46:1–2

32c. Mendenhall C, Roselle G, et al 1986 *False-Positive Tests for HTLV-III [HIV] Antibodies in Alcoholic Patients with Hepatitis* NEJM 314:921

33c. Moore J, Cone E, et al 1986 *HTLV-III [HIV] Seropositivity in 1971–1972 Parenteral Drug Abusers: A Case of False-Positives or Evidence of Viral Exposure?* NEJM 314:1387–1388

34c. Mortimer P, Mortimer J, et al 1985 *Which Anti-HTLV-III/LAV [HIV] Assays for Screening and Confirmatory Testing?* Lancet October 19, p873

35c. Neale T, Dagger J, et al 1985 *False-Positive Anti-HTLV-III [HIV] Serology* New Zealand Med J October 23

36c. Ng V 1991 *Serological Diagnosis with Recombinant Peptides/Proteins* Clin Chem 37:1667–1668

37c. Ozanne G, Fauvel M 1988 *Performance and Reliability of Five Commercial Enzyme-Linked Immunosorbent Assay Kits in Screening for Anti-Human Immunodeficiency Virus Antibody in High-Risk Subjects* J Clin Micro 26:1496

38c. Papadopulos-Eleopulos E 1988 *Reappraisal of AIDS: Is the Oxidation Induced by the Risk Factors the Primary Cause?* Med Hypo 25:151

39c. Papadopulos-Eleopulos E, Turner V, et al 1993 *Is a Positive Western Blot Proof of HIV Infection?* Bio/Technology June 11:696–707

40c. Pearlman ES, Ballas SK 1994 *False-Positive Human Immunodeficiency Virus Screening Test Related to Rabies Vaccination* Arch Pathol Lab Med 118–805

41c. Peternan T, Lang G, et al 1986 *Hemodialysis/Renal Failure* JAMA 255:2324

42c. Piszkewicz D 1987 *HTLV-III [HIV] Antibodies after Immune Globulin* JAMA 257:316

43c. Profitt M, Yen-Lieberman B 1993 *Laboratory Diagnosis of Human Immunodeficiency Virus Infection* Inf Dis Clin North Am 7:203

44c. Ranki A, Kurki P, et al 1992 *Antibodies to Retroviral Proteins in Autoimmune Connective Tissue Disease* Arthritis and Rheumatism 35:1483

45c. Ribeiro T, Brites C, et al 1993 *Serologic Validation of HIV Infection in a Tropical Area* JAIDS 6:319

46c. Sayers M, Beatty P, et al 1986 *HLA Antibodies as a Cause of False-Positive Reactions in Screening Enzyme Immunoassays for Antibodies to Human T-Lymphotropic Virus Type III [HIV]* Transfusion 26(1):114

47c. Sayre K, Dodd R, et al 1996 *False-Positive Human Immunodeficiency Virus Type 1 Western Blot Tests in Non-Infected Blood Donors* Transfusion 36:45

48c. Schleupner C *Detection of HIV-1 infection* In: Principles and Practice of Infectious Diseases, 3rd ed. by Mandell G, Douglas R, Bennett J (eds.) Churchill Livingstone, New York 1990:1092

49c. Schochetman G, George J 1992 *Serologic Tests for the Detection of Human Immunodeficiency Virus Infection* AIDS Testing: Methodology and Management Issues, Springer-Verlag, New York

50c. Simonsen L, Buffington J, et al 1995 *Multiple False Reactions in Viral Antibody Screening Assays after Influenza Vaccination* Am J Epide. 141–1089

51c. Smith D, Dewhurst S, et al 1987 *False-Positive Enzyme-Linked Immunosorbent Assay Reactions for Antibody to Human Immunodeficiency Virus in a Population of Midwestern Patients with Congenital Bleeding Disorders* Transfusion 127:112

52c. Snyder H, Fleissner E 1980 *Specificity of Human Antibodies to Oncovirus Glycoproteins* Proc Natl Acad Sci 77:1622–1626

53c. Steckelberg J, Cockerill F 1988 *Serologic Testing for Human Immunodeficiency Virus Antibodies* Mayo Clin Proc 63:373

54c. Sungar C, Akpolat T, et al *Alpha Interferon Therapy in Hemodialysis Patients* Nephron 67:251

55c. Tribe D, Reed D, et al 1988 *Antibodies Reactive with Human Immunodeficiency Virus Gag-Coated Antigens (Gag Reactive Only) are a Major Cause of Enzyme-Linked Immunosorbent Assay Reactivity in a Blood Donor Population* J Clin Micro April:641

56c. Ujhelyi E, Fust G, et al 1989 *Different Types of False Positive Anti-HIV Reactions in Patients on Hemodialysis* Immun Let 22:35–40

57c. Van Beers D, Duys M, et al *Heat Inactivation of Serum May Interfere with Tests for Antibodies to LAV/HTLV-III [HIV]* J Vir Meth 12:329

58c. Voevodin A 1992 *HIV Screening in Russia* Lancet 339:1548

59c. Weber B, Moshtaghi-Borojeni M, et al 1995 *Evaluation of the Reliability of Six Current Anti-HIV-1/HIV-2 Enzyme Immunoassays* J Vir Meth 55:97

60c. Wood C, Williams A, et al 1986 *Antibody Against the Human Immunodeficiency Virus in Commercial Intravenous Gammaglobulin Preparations* Ann Int Med 105:536

61c. Yale S, Degroen P, et al 1994 *Unusual Aspects of Acute Q Fever-Associated Hepatitis* Mayo Clin Proc 69:769

62c. Yoshida T, Matsui T, et al 1987 *Evaluation of Passive Particle Agglutination Test for Antibody to Human Immunodeficiency Virus* J Clin Micro Aug:1433

63c. Yu S, Fong C, et al 1989 *A False Positive HIV Antibody Reaction Due to Transfusion-Induced HLA-DR4 Sensitization* NEJM 320:1495

64c. National Institute of Justice *AIDS Bulletin* October 1988

33. Curran J 1985 *The Epidemiology of AIDS: Current Status and Future Prospects* Science 229:1352–1357; Karon, et al 1996 *Prevalence of HIV Infections in the US* Journal of the American Medical Association 276:126–131; Krieger L *One in 300 US Adults Infected,* San Francisco Examiner July 7 1996 pA82

34. NBC Nightly News, March 10 1995: Robert Hager of NBC reported that the CDC was about to lower estimates they knew were too high. CDC spokesperson Michelle Bond remarked that the CDC officials were reluctant to report lower numbers for fear of adverse budgetary consequences.

35. All STDs except genital herpes: US Centers for Disease Control 1997, Table 1: Cases of STDs reported by state health departments in US 1941–1997, STD Surveillance p65–66. Genital herpes: Meyer T March 24 1998 Associated Press, Atlanta (Meyer quotes CDC and Dr. Charles Bell of Texas Department of Health)

36. US Centers for Disease Control 1999 *HIV/AIDS Surveillance Report* Year-end edition 1998 (Deaths in persons with AIDS, cumulative totals through December 1998) Table 21, p30

37. US Centers for Disease Control 1998 *HIV/AIDS Surveillance Report* Year-end edition 1997 (US HIV and AIDS cases reported through December 1997) Table 13 states "Reported deaths are not necessarily caused by HIV-related disease"

38. CDC Wonder website; The New York Times, death count, all ages, all races, both genders 1981–1998

39. Lazarou J, et al 1998 *Incidence of Adverse Drug Reactions in Hospitalized Patients (1966–1996)* Journal of the American Medical Association, 279:1200; Manmaney T *Medications Kill 100,000 Annually* Los Angeles Times April 15 1998

40. PBS 1998 The American Experience: Influenza 1918

41. World Health Organization *Weekly Epidemiological Record* November 1999

42. UNAIDS 1999 *World AIDS Campaign Facts and Figures*; World Health Organization June 1998, *Weekly Epidemiological Record*

43. *CDC National Vital Statistics Report* October 7 1998, Vol 47:4 Table E p7 (Deaths and death rates, final 1996 and preliminary 1997)

44. Geshekter C 1997 *AIDS: The Leading Cause of Unjustified Hysteria,* Reappraising AIDS, February Vol 5:2

45. Institute of Medicine (IOM) 1996 *Scientific Opportunities and Public Needs*; Webster K *Disproportionate Funding* Associated Press June 16 1999

46. US Centers for Disease Control 1999 *HIV/AIDS Surveillance Report* Year-end edition 1998

47. Crowne D, et al 1964 *The Approval Motive* John Wiley and Sons, New York; Saxe L 1991 *Lying: Thoughts of an Applied Social Psychologist* American Psychologist 46:409–415; Source: Brody S *Sex at Risk* Transaction Publishers, New Brunswick

48. Brody, S 1997 *Sex at Risk* Transaction Publishers, New Brunswick; 80%: Potterat, et al 1987 JAMA 256 p 12; 65%: Renzullo, et al 1990 JAIDS 3, p266–271; 83%–90%: Committee on AIDS Research and the Behavioral, Social, and Statistical Sciences 1989; 69%: Chicago Dept of Public Health, Journal of AIDS 1997; 99.4%: NYC Dept of Health, American Journal of Epidemiology 137:2

49. Figures for AIDS by Risk Groups are based on cumulative figures through 1998 and do not include cases where risk status was not assessed; AIDS by Health Status are for years 1993 through 1997 using Table 11 of the 93–97 US CDC HIV/AIDS Surveillance Reports (1997 was the last year the CDC published the data in Table 11); AIDS by Gender is based on cumulative figures through 1998

50. US Centers for Disease Control 1999 *HIV/AIDS Surveillance Report* Year-end 1998

51. Burke D, et al 1990 *Seroprevalence Among Applicants for US Military Service* Unpublished data through 1997 from US Military Processing: For a copy of this unpublished data, send a SASE to the author

52. US Centers for Disease Control 1999 *HIV/AIDS Surveillance Report* Year-end 1998 p26

53. Duesberg P 1996 *Inventing the AIDS Virus* Regnery Press, Washington DC p183

54. Holding R, Carlsen W 1998 *Epidemic Ravages Caregivers* San Francisco Chronicle p1, A6–A8

55. US Centers for Disease Control 1999 *HIV/AIDS Surveillance Report* Year-end 1998 Table 7 p14; US Centers for Disease Control 1998 HIV/AIDS Surveillance Report Year-end 1997 Table 8 p15
56. Laboratory Centre for Disease Control, Health Canada, April 1998 *Gonorrhea in Canada*; US Centers for Disease Control 1998 *HIV/AIDS Surveillance Report* Year-end 1997, Tables 13A and 13B; Interview with LCDC Bureau of AIDS and STDs Office of Don Sutherland, September 14, 1998: Gonorrhea cases in Canada
57. US Centers for Disease Control 1999 *HIV/AIDS Surveillance Report* Year-end 1998 Table 7 p14; US Centers for Disease Control 1998 *HIV/AIDS Surveillance Report* Year-end 1997 Table 8 p15
58. Mok, et al 1987 *Infants Born to Mothers Seropositive for HIV* Lancet 1164–1168; European Collaborative Study 1991 *Children Born to Women with HIV 1* Lancet 337:253–260
59. Source: National Center for Health Statistics July 1996 703/821-8955: Cumulative SIDS deaths in children under 1 year of age 1983–1996, 1997 preliminary, 1981–1982 computed by average of years 1983–1993
60. Transactions of the Society of Actuaries, Vol XLIV p333–97; Boffey P April 22 1988, *Researchers List Odds of Getting AIDS in Heterosexual Intercourse* New York Times; Hearst N, Hulley S April 1988 Journal of the American Medical Association; *Dangers Real and Imagined* December 8 1997 Wall Street Journal; Discover magazine, May 1996 p82
61. World Health Organization, November 1999 *Weekly Epidemiological Record*
62. Harvard University Global Burden of Disease Study, 1996; World Health Organization, Geneva 1996 *Fighting Disease, Fostering Development*; Geshekter C *Rethinking AIDS in Africa* Reappraising AIDS Vol 3:2 February 1995
63. World Health Organization 1985 Bangui definition for AIDS in Africa (in current use); WHO case definitions for AIDS surveillance in adults and adolescents *Weekly Epidemiological Record* September 1994 69:273–80 (confirmed April 1999 by WHO)
64. World Health Organization, November 1999 *Weekly Epidemiological Record (current)*; Harvard University Global Burden of Disease Study, 1996; World Health Organization, Geneva 1996 *Fighting Disease, Fostering Development*; Geshekter C *Rethinking AIDS in Africa* Reappraising AIDS Vol 3:2 February 1995; World Health Organization 1985 Bangui definition for AIDS in Africa (in current use); WHO case definitions for AIDS surveillance in adults and adolescents *Weekly Epidemiological Record* September 1994 69:273–80 (confirmed April 1999 by WHO); World Health Organization *World Health Report 1998* Annual cases of selected diseases
65. Kestler H, et al 1990 *Induction of AIDS in Rhesus Monkey by Molecularly Cloned SIV* Science 2448:1109–112; Kestler, et al 1991 *Importance of Net Gene for Maintenance of High Virus Loads* Cell 65:651–662; Fultz, et al 1990 *Humoral Response to SIV/SMM Infection in Macaque and Mangabey Monkeys* Journal of AIDS 3:319–329; Weiss R, et al 1985 *Molecular Biology of RNA Tumor Viruses* Cold Spring Harbor Press, New York; Blatner W, et al 1988 *HIV Causes AIDS* Science 241:514–515; Lambrou E 1994 *AIDS Scare or Scam* p14–15 Vantage Press, New York
66. Gao, et al *Nature* February 4 1999
67. World Health Organization, *Weekly Epidemiological Record,* November 26 1999
68. Russell R *Kenya Slow to Face Up to AIDS Scourge* Reuters November 25 1998
69. World Health Organization *World Health Report 1998*; *Weekly Epidemiological Record,* November 26 1999
70. World Health Organization *World Health Report 1998* Annual cases of selected diseases
71. Journal of AIDS 1994 7:8 p876
72. US Centers for Disease Control 1999 *HIV/AIDS Surveillance Report* Year-end 1998; 9(2) Calculations: David Crowe, Alberta Reappraising AIDS Society
73. US Centers for Disease Control *HIV/AIDS Surveillance Report* Year-end editions 1997, 1996, 1995, 1994, 1993 (AIDS indicator conditions reported by age group, United States)
74. US Centers for Disease Control 1998 *HIV/AIDS Surveillance Report* Year-end 1997 p25 Figure 6
75. US Centers for Disease Control 1998 *HIV/AIDS Surveillance Report* Year-end 1997 p25 Figure 6
76. POZ magazine July 1999: Glaxo-Wellcome Ad for Ziagen (abacavir sulfate), December 1998 MG-001; Merck Ad for Crixivan (indinavir) Merck and Co, Inc. 1998 99-4084; Roxanne Ad for Viramune (nevirapine) July 1999, RX-2140 (4/98); Glaxo-Wellcome Ad for Combivir (lamivudine/zidovudine) March 1999
77. POZ magazine July 1999: Glaxo-Wellcome Ad for Combivir
78. Hammer S, et al 1997 *A Controlled Trial of Two Nucleoside Analogues Indinavir in Persons with HIV* New England Journal of Medicine 337:725–733
79. Merck Ad for Crixivan (indinavir) Merck and Co, Inc. 1998 99-4084
80. POZ magazine July 1999: Glaxo-Wellcome Ad for Ziagen (abacavir sulfate), December 1998 MG-001; Merck Ad for Crixivan (indinavir) Merck and Co, Inc. 1998 99-4084; Roxanne Ad for Viramune (nevirapine) July 1999, RX-2140 (4/98); Glaxo-Wellcome Ad for Combivir (lamivudine/zidovudine), March 1999; FDA Advisory (warning of spontaneous bleeding in 15 hemophiliacs using protease inhibitors), July 16 1996; Dube M, Johnson D, et al 1997 Protease *Inhibitor Associated Hyperglycemia* Lancet 350:713–4; Kotler D *Truncal Obesity* February 20 1998 Clinical Care Options for HIV (Monthly Experts Column); Garrett L *The Virus at the End of the World* Esquire March 1 1999; Lo J, et al 1998 *Buffalo Hump in Men with HIV-1* Lancet March 21 1998 p867–870; Miller KD, et al *Visceral Abdominal Fat Accumulation Associated with Use of Indinavir* p871–875; Kim L *FDA Approves Another Protease Inhibitor* The Atlanta Journal and Constitution April 17 1999 p2E; Mickleburgh R, *Study AIDS Drugs Long Term, Makers Told* The Globe and Mail (Canada) May 4 1999; Colebunders E, et al *Sexual Dysfunction with Protease Inhibitors* Lancet 353 May 22 1999; Waldholz M, Tanouye E *Cocktail Break* Wall Street Journal January 25 1999
81. Staszewski S et al 1999 *Efavirenz plus Zidovudine and Lamivudine in the Treatment of HIV-1 Infection in Adults*, New England Journal of Medicine Vol 341, No 25; December 3 1999 2:37 AM EST PlanetOut: Community Headlines AIDS: Current Global Numbers; James Curran on CNN, August 23 1998 8:00 PM EST
82. Altman L *New Cases Widen Views About AIDS* New York Times January 5 1984
83. Auberbach, et al 1984, Am J Med 76:487; Boffey P *AIDS in the Future: Risk of Developing AIDS* New York Times January 14 1986; JAMA 262: 3129–3130; Burkett E *HIV: Not Guilty?* Miami Herald December 23 1990 p12–17
84. Eckholm E *Onset of AIDS After Transfusion Found to Lag Average of 5 Years,* New York Times May 29 1986; Lambrou E 1994 *AIDS: Scare or Scam?* Vantage Press, New York p15; Garrett L June 1999 *Blacks May Have Genetic Risk of HIV Infection*, Alive & Kicking!; Waldholz M, Tanouye E *Cocktail Break* Wall Street Journal January 25 1999
85. Johnson C, Philpott P *Viral Load of Crap* Reappraising AIDS Vol 4:10 October 1996; Duesberg P 1995 Nature 357 p197

86. Rasnick D *Kinetics Analysis of Consecutive HIV Proteolytic Cleavages of the Gag-Pol Polyprotein* Journal of Biological Chemistry March 7 1997
87. Mullis K October 1998 *The Medical Establishment vs. The Truth* Penthouse Magazine
88. Rich J, et al 1999 *Misdiagnosis of HIV Infection by HIV-1 Plasma Viral Load Testing: A Case Series* Annals of Internal Medicine 130:37–39; Sullivan, et al *Persistently Negative HIV-1 Antibody Enzyme Immunoassay Screening Results for Patients with HIV-1 Infection and AIDS* AIDS January 14 1999 13:89–96
89. Piatak M March 19 1993 *High Levels of HIV-1 in Plasma During All Stages of Infection Determined by Competitive PCR* Science 259:1749–53; Roehr B *Loading Zone* POZ Magazine August 1999 p76
90. New England Journal of Medicine November 3 1994 331:18 p1176–1177
91. Semba R, et al 1993 *Increased Mortality Associated with Vitamin A Deficiency During HIV-1 Infection* Arch Intern Med 153:2149-2154
92. WHO/UNAIDS, 1998 *HIV and Infant Feeding: A Guide for Health Care Managers and Supervisors* FRH/Nut 98, 22
93. *HealthNews* Mothering magazine Summer 1997 p40; Dew J October 8 1999 *Newborn HIV Tests Criticized* New Haven Register
94. Farber C *AZT Roulette: The Impossible Choices Facing HIV Positive Mothers* Mothering magazine September/October 1998 Issue 90
95. Semba R, et al 1993 *Increased Mortality Associated with Vitamin A Deficiency During HIV-1 Infection* Arch Intern Med 153:2149–2154
96. Kumar R, et al 1994 *Zidovudine Use in Pregnancy: A Report on 104 cases and Birth Defects* Journal of AIDS 7(10):1034–1039
97. Cordes R, et al 1995 *Pitfalls in HIV Testing* Postgraduate Medicine 98:177; Ng V, et al *Serological Diagnosis with Recombinant Peptides/Proteins* Clinical Chemistry 37:1667–1668; Profitt M, et al 1993 *Laboratory Diagnosis of HIV Infection* Inf Dis Clin North Am 7:203; Steckelberg J, Cockerill F 1988 *Serologic Testing for HIV Antibodies* Mayo Clinic Proc 63:373; Voevodi A 1992 *HIV Screening in Russia* Lancet 339:1548
98. Mothering magazine Summer 1997 *Health News* p40
99. Cleary, et al 1987 Journal of the American Medical Association 258(13):1757–62
100. US Centers for Disease Control *Recommendations of the US Public Heath Service Task Force on the Use of Zidovudine [AZT] to Reduce Perinatal Transmission of HIV* Morbidity and Mortality Weekly Report Vol 43 No RR-11 August 5 1994
101. Regush N *No AZT For My Baby, Please* ABCNews.com September 16 1999
102. Gwarteny D *Baby's Risk for HIV Sparks Fight* The Oregonian January 31 1999; Wright J *Court Grants Delay in Baby HIV Case* The Register-Guard February 5 1999
103. Good Morning America September 9 1998
104. Philpott P *Maine Mother Wins Court Fight Against HIV Doctors* Reappraising AIDS Vol 6 October 10 1998
105. *Mother Wins Right to Stop HIV Drugs* New York Times April 20 1999; Dateline NBC January 25, 1999; *A Mother's Instinct* People Magazine October 5 1998 p157–158
106. News Broadcast, CJOB 68 August 18 1999; Peritz I *Mother Fights to Block Son's HIV Drug Therapy* The Globe and Mail (Canada) August 18 1999
107. McKittrick A *Ethical Drug Pricing: An Oxymoron?* Provincetown Positive Spring 1999 p37–39
108. Duesberg P 1996 *Inventing the AIDS Virus* Regnery Press, Washington DC p 309–359
109. *Physicians Desk Reference* 1994 p32
110. Duesberg P 1996 *Inventing the AIDS Virus* Regnery Press, Washington DC p 309–359
111. Lauritsen J 1993 *The AIDS War* Askelpios, New York, FDA Documents Show Fraud in AZT Trials p381–397
112. Lancet 1993 343:871, Concorde Coordinating Committee; Journal of the American Medical Association 1988 203:3009; New England Journal of Medicine 1992 326:437. Source: Hand T *Why Antiviral Drugs Cannot Resolve AIDS* Reappraising AIDS Vol 4:9 September 1996
113. Source: Interview with Dr. Charles Thomas in video HIV=AIDS: Fact or Fraud? Starvision Productions (Stephen Allen, prod.) Denver CO; Duesberg P 1996 *Inventing the AIDS Virus* Regnery Press, Washington DC p 309–359
114. British Medical Journal July 15 1995 p156–158 (49%); Science Magazine February 24 1995 p1080 (34%); JAMA 260:3009 1988; New England Journal of Medicine 1992, 326:437. Source: Hand T *Why Antiviral Drugs Cannot Resolve AIDS* Reappraising AIDS Vol 4:9 September 1996
115. Merck Manual 1992 16th edition p55, Merck Research Laboratories; Glaxo-Wellcome information sheet accompanying Zidovudine
116. Hammer S, et al 1997 *A Controlled Trial of Two Nucleoside Analogues Indinavir in Persons with HIV* New England Journal of Medicine 337:725–733
117. Merck ad for Crixivan A&U magazine July 1999 99-4084 910 (508) CRX
118. Anderson M *The Big Tease* Valley Advocate February 20 1997
119. Interview with Christine Maggiore September 1997
120. AIDS expert Dr. Bruce Walker on ABC News Nightline May 19 1999 11:35 PM EST
121. Ostrom N The New York Native July 15 1996 Issue 691
122. POZ magazine July 1999: Glaxo-Wellcome Ad for Ziagen (abacavir sulfate), December 1998 MG-001; Merck Ad for Crixivan (indinavir) Merck and Co, Inc. 1998 99-4084; Roxanne Ad for Viramune (nevirapine) July 1999, RX-2140 (4/98); Glaxo-Wellcome Ad for Combivir (lamivudine/zidovudine) March 1999
123. Journal of the American Medical Association July 10 1996
124. Johnson H Rolling Stone Magazine *Special Report: Dr. David Ho and the Lazarus Equation* March 6 1997
125. Levy J 1996 *AIDS Surrogate Markers: Is There Truth in Numbers?* JAMA Vol 276 p161–162
126. Merck ad for Crixivan A&U magazine July 1999 99-4084 910 (508) CRX
127. Altman L New York Times February 2 1996; Garrett L Newsday March 5 1996; The Boston Globe February 1 1999
128. Dr. Raymond Schinazi of Emory University, Atlanta, Georgia. Source: Garrett L Newsday March 31 1995
129. Lancet June 1 1997 Vol 349 p1745; Associated Press Report, Philadelphia Inquirer June 13 1997; Anderson M *The Big Tease* The Valley Advocate February 20 1997; Green F *Cocktail Hangover* Cleveland Free Times May 5 1999 Vol 7 Issue 33; Signorile M *641,086 and Counting* Out magazine September 1998
130. *The Morning After* POZ magazine February 1997
131. US Centers for Disease Control 1999 *HIV/AIDS Surveillance Report* Year-end 1998; 9(2) Calculations: David Crowe, Alberta Reappraising AIDS Society; US Centers for Disease Control 1998 *HIV/AIDS Surveillance Report* Year-end 1997 p25 Figure 6
132. US Centers for Disease Control *HIV/AIDS Surveillance Report* Year-end editions 1997, 1996, 1995, 1994, 1993 (AIDS indicator conditions reported by age group, US)

133. Interview with Christine Maggiore September 1997

134. Janeway C, Travers P, et al 1999 *Immunobiology: The Immune System in Health and Disease*, 4th edition, Elsevier Science Ltd/Garland Publishing, New York; Pizzo PA 1999 *Fever in Immunocompromised Patients*, New England Journal of Medicine 16;341:893–900; Sussman E September 1999 *Fat Disorders: A Growing Threat, Health Risks Include Heart Disease*, HIVPlus, No 5, http://www.aegis.com/pubs/hivplus/1999/sep/fat.html; Peto T, May 1996, *Surrogate Markers in HIV Disease*, Journal of Antimicrobial Chemotherapy 37(B):161–170

135. Gallo R 1984 Science 224; Piatak M 1993 Science 259; Ho D 1991 New England Journal of Medicine 324:961; Shaw G 1991 New England Journal of Medicine 324:954; Cooper 1992 Lancet 341:1099

136. Duesberg P 1996 *Inventing the AIDS Virus* Regnery Press, Washington DC p174–180

137. Bialy H, Duesberg P March 1995 Letter to Nature. Source: *AIDS: Virus or Drug Induced?* Duesberg P (editor) 1996 Kluwer Academic Publishers, Netherlands

138. Ho D, et al 1995 *Rapid Turnover of Plasma Virions and CD4 Lymphocytes in HIV-1 Infection* Nature 373:123–126; Wei X, et al 1995 Nature 373:117–122

139. Kary Mullis at HEAL Los Angeles, October 25 1995

140. Philpott P, Johnson C 1996 *Viral Load of Crap* Reappraising AIDS Vol 4:10 p2

141. Johnson C *Viral Load and the PCR* Continuum Vol 4:4 November/ December 1996

142. CDC faxback document #320320 sent in reply to an inquiry by Christine Johnson

143. Roche Amplicor PCR Diagnostics HIV-1 Monitor test kit pamphlet

144. Defer C, et al 1992 *Multicenter Quality Control of PCR Detection of HIV DNA* AIDS 6:659–663; Bush, et al 1992, Journal of AIDS 5:872; Gerberding J 1994 *Incidence and Prevalence of HIV, Hepatitis B, and CMV Among Health Care Personnel at Risk for Blood Exposure* Journal of Infectious Disease 170:1410–1417; de Mendoza, et al 1998 *False Positive for HIV Using Commercial Viral Load Quantification Assays* AIDS 12:2076–2077; Rich J, et al 1999 *Misdiagnosis of HIV Infection by HIV-1 Plasma Viral Load Testing: A Case Series*, Annals of Internal Medicine 130:37–39

145. Schwartz D, et al 1997 *Extensive Evaluation of a Seronegative Participant in an HIV-1 Vaccine Trial as a Result of False-Positive PCR*, Lancet Vol 350 No 9073 p256

146. Rasnick D 1997 *Kinetics Analysis of Consecutive HIV Proteolytic Cleavages of the Gag-Pol Polyprotein* Journal of Biological Chemistry March 7 p6348–6353

147. Piatak M, et al 1993 Science 259:1749–53

148. Roderer M 1998 *Getting to the HAART of T Cell Dynamics* Nature Medicine Vol 4:2 p145–146; Levy J 1996 *AIDS Surrogate Markers: Is There Truth in Numbers?* JAMA Vol 276 p161–162

149. Levy J 1996 *AIDS Surrogate Markers: Is There Truth in Numbers?* JAMA Vol 276 p161–162

150. Philpott P, Johnson C 1996 *Viral Load of Crap* Reappraising AIDS Vol 4:10 p2

151. Papadopulos-Eleopulos E, et al 1988 *Reappraisal of AIDS: Is the Oxidation Induced by the Risk Factors the Primary Cause?* Medical Hypothesis 25:151–162

152. Papadopulos-Eleopulos E, et al 1993 *Is A Positive Western Blot Proof of HIV Infection?* Bio/Technology 11:696–707; Papadopulos-Eleopulos E, et al 1996 *The Isolation of HIV: Has it Really Been Achieved?* Continuum Vol 4:3 Supplement p1–24; Turner V 1996 *Do HIV Antibody Tests Prove HIV Infection?* Continuum 1996 Vol 3:5 p8–11; Papadopulos-Eleopulos E, Stewart G, et al 1997 *HIV Antibodies: Further Questions and a Plea for Clarification* Current Medical Research and Opinion 13:627–634

153. Philpott P 1997 *The Isolation Question* Reappraising AIDS Vol 5:6 June/July/August

154. Gallo R 1984 Science 224:497–508; Piatak M 1993 Science 259:1749–1754; Piatak M 1993 Lancet 341:1099; Daar, et al 1991 New England Journal of Medicine 324[14]:961–964; Clark, et al 1991 New England Journal of Medicine 324:954–960; Cooper, et al 1992 Lancet 340:1257–1258

155. Nature Magazine May 26 1994

156. *Morning Report* Los Angeles Times May 16 1996 F-2

157. Project Inform letter to Dr. Bruce Alberts, President of the National Academy of Sciences, July 31 1997: Endorsements are for signers as of August 20 1997

158. Letter to Christine Maggiore from Ric Parish, PLUS Programs Manager, May 30 1997

159. Anderson MK 1997 *Sick of It All* The Valley Advocate January 15 1998

160. Farber C 1995 *AIDS Inc.: Observations of an AIDS Dissident* Provincetown Positive April/May Issue p14–18

161. Garrett L *The Virus at the End of The World* Esquire magazine March 1999

162. A&U America's AIDS Magazine June 1999 Issue 56

163. Duesberg P 1987 *Retroviruses as Carcinogens and Pathogens: Expectations and Reality* Cancer Research 47:1199–1220

164. Interview with Christine Maggiore August 25 1999

165. Eichenwald K, Kolata G *Drug Trials Hide Conflicts for Doctors* New York Times May 16 1999

166. Smith M, *Sticking Point: AIDS Vaccine Designed by Don Francis in Final Testing* San Francisco Weekly July 14 1999

167. CNN Website *Massive Trial of AIDS Vaccine to Begin in Thailand* February 10 1999 8:27 pm EST

168. *Dissecting Room* Lancet Vol 353 May 15 1999 p1719

169. McGinley L *Price of Success: Powerful Treatments Create Growing Rift Among AIDS Groups* Wall Street Journal December 20 1996

170. *Drug Money* Counter Punch magazine July 1 1998

171. Farber C 1995 *AIDS Inc.: Observations of an AIDS Dissident* Provincetown Positive April/May Issue p14–18

172. US Centers for Disease Control *HIV/AIDS Surveillance Report* Year-end editions through 1998

173. WHO website *http://hivinsite.ucsf.edu/social/un/2098.3ce6.html* Ratios of estimated AIDS cases/reported AIDS cases for African countries with highest estimated AIDS cases: Angola 22/1; Congo 13/1; Ethiopia 55/1; Kenya 9/1; Madagascar 69/1; Mozambique 48/1; Nigeria 35/1; South Africa 33/1; Uganda 37/1; Zimbabwe 10/1. For all African countries (with available data) combined, the ratio of estimated AIDS cases to reported AIDS cases is 16/1

174. CDC national AIDS advertising campaign, October 1987: 38 TV commercials, 8 radio spots, 6 print ads

175. Bennett A, Sharpe A *Health Hazard: AIDS Fight Skewed by Federal Campaign Exaggerating Risks* Wall Street Journal May 1996 p1

176. Philpott P *CDC Releases Data for 1995: What HIV/AIDS Epidemic?* Reappraising AIDS Vol 4:7 July 1996

177. US Centers for Disease Control *HIV/AIDS Surveillance Report* Year-end editions 1993 through 1998 with one exception: AIDS in teenage boys rose from 238 in 1994 to 245 in 1995

178. Laboratory Centre for Disease Control, Health Canada, 1998 *HIV and AIDS in Canada: Surveillance Report to December 31 1997* p1

179. Until There's a Cure advertisement *www.until.org*

180. Interview with Patty Dwyer from Until There's A Cure September 3, 1999 (800) 888-UNTIL

181. WHO website *http://hivinsite.ucsf.edu/social/un/2098.3ce6.html* Ratios of estimated AIDS cases/reported AIDS cases for African countries with highest estimated AIDS cases: Angola 22/1; Congo 13/1; Ethiopia 55/1; Kenya 9/1; Madagascar 69/1; Mozambique 48/1; Nigeria 35/1; South Africa 33/1; Uganda 37/1; Zimbabwe 10/1. For all African countries (with available data) combined, the ratio of estimated AIDS cases to reported AIDS cases is 16/1

182. *China Says HIV Cases Estimated at 400,000* April 1 1999 4:25 am EST Reuters, Bejing

183. *Merck Manual* 1899 first edition

184. Mendelsohn R 1984 *How To Raise a Healthy Child In Spite of Your Doctor* Ballentine Books, New York p13–15

185. *The American Medical Association Encyclopedia of Medicine* Random House, New York p359; Mendelsohn R 1979 *Confessions of a Medical Heretic* Contemporary Publishing Company, Chicago p28–29

186. *The American Medical Association Encyclopedia of Medicine* 1989 Random House, New York p 977

187. Kono R 1975 *The SMON Virus Theory* Lancet ii:370–371; Shigematsu H, et al 1975 *Epidemiological Approach to SMON* Japanese Journal of Medicine, Science and Biology, 28 Supplement 23–33; Soda T 1980 *Drug Induced Sufferings: Medical, Pharmaceutical and Legal Aspects* Excerpta Medica: Amersterdam

188. Marshall B *Why Doctors Aren't Curing Ulcers* Fortune Magazine June 9 1997

189. Haney D *Doctors Slow to Attack Bug Behind Ulcers* Los Angeles Times (API) February 11 1996

190. Marshall B *Why Doctors Aren't Curing Ulcers* Fortune Magazine June 9 1997

191. NIAID and NIH Report 1996 *The Relationship Between HIV and AIDS* p3

192. Giraldo R 1997 *AIDS and Stressors* Fundacion Arte y Cincia, Medellin; Root-Bernstein R 1993 *Rethinking AIDS* The Free Press, New York; Al Bayati A 1999 *Get All the Facts: HIV Does Not Cause AIDS* Toxi-Health, Dixon, CA

193. Root-Bernstein R 1993 *Rethinking AIDS* The Free Press, New York p220–280; Brody S 1997 *Sex at Risk* Transaction Publishers, New Brunswick; Plumley P 1995 *Condomania: Common Sense or Nonsense?* HEAL Bulletin, HEAL New York

194. Willner R 1994 *Deadly Deception* p30 Peltec Publishing; *The Merck Manual* 1992 Immunodeficiency Diseases p303 Table 19-1 Merck Research Laboratories, Rahway; Fauci A, et al 1998 *Principles of Internal Medicine, Edition 14* McGraw Hill, New York

195. Chandra R 1983 *Nutrition, Immunity and Infection* Lancet i:688–69. Source: *AIDS and Stressors*; *Merck Manual* 1992 Immunodeficiency Diseases p317–318, Immunodeficiency and Malnutrition Merck Research Laboratories, Rahway; Chandra R 1975 *Fetal Malnutrition and Postnatal Immunocompetence* American Journal of Dis Chil 125:450–455. Source: *AIDS and Stressors*

196. *Merck Manual* 1992 Immunodeficiency Diseases, p304 Table 19-2 Immunosuppressive Agents Merck Research Laboratories, Rahway; Heyer A 1983 *Introduction to Nutrition* Keats Publishing, New Canaan p2–12; Owen B 1995 *You Don't Have to Die Sick* Adrenal Exhaustion p43–46 Health Hope Publishing House, Cannon Beach

197. *The American Medical Association Encyclopedia of Medicine* 1989 Random House, New York p258

198. Niwa Y, Yokoyama M 1981 *Effect of Glucocorticosteroid Therapy on the Immune System of Patients with Nonimmunologically Mediated Dermatose* J Clin Lab Immunol 6(2):147–155; Parrillo J, Fauci A 1978 *Mechanisms of Corticosteroid Action on Lymphocyte Subpopulations of Effector Cells Mediating Cellular Toxicity in Man* Clin Exp Immunol 31:116–125; Fauci A. Dale D, Balow J 1976 *Glucocorticosteroid Therapy: Mechanisms of Action and Clinical Considerations* Annals of Internal Medicine 84:304–15; Leung F, Fam A, Osoba D 1981 *Kaposi's Sarcoma Complicating Corticosteroid Therapy for Temporal Arteritis* The American Journal of Medicine 71(2):320–322

199. *Merck Manual* 1992 Anti-Infective Drugs: Sulfonamides p46–48 Merck Research Laboratories, Rahway; *Drugs Facts and Comparisons* 1999 Facts and Comparisons Publishing, St. Louis (800) 223-0554

200. Duesberg P 1996 *Inventing The AIDS Virus* Regnery Publishing, Washington DC p300

201. *Merck Manual* 1992 Anti-Infective Drugs: Sulfonamides p46–48 Merck Research Laboratories, Rahway; *Drugs Facts and Comparisons* 1999 Facts and Comparisons Publishing, St. Louis (800) 223-0554

202. Bull Mem Soc Med Hopitaux de Paris, 3rd Ser 1909, 28:958–996; Pharmacology Ther 1992 55: 201–207

203. *Immune System Toxins* Rachel's Environment and Health Weekly #536 March 6 1997; *Statement on Immune Toxins* #544 May 1 1997 Environmental Research Foundation, Annapolis

204. Hebert C, Brecher M, et al *Fewer Blood Transfusions Save Lives* New England Journal of Medicine February 1999; United Press International, February 10 1999; Ward, et al 1989 *The Natural History of Transfusion Associated Infection With HIV* New England Journal of Medicine 321:947–952

205. Benson H 1997 *The Nocebo Effect: History and Physiology* Preventive Medicine 26:612–615; Binik Y 1985 *Psychosocial Predictors of Sudden Death: A Review and Critique* Social Science Medicine 20(7):667–80; Cecchi R 1984 *Stress: Prodrome to Immune Deficiency* Annals of the New York Academy of Sciences 437:286–289; Cohen S 1988 *Voodoo Death, the Stress Response, and AIDS* Advanced Biochem Psychopharmacology 44:95–109; Golden K *Voodoo in Africa and the United States* December 1977 American Journal of Psychiatry 134 (12):1425–1427; Uno H, et al 1989 *Hippocampal Damage Associated with Prolonged and Fatal Stress in Primates* Journal of Neuroscience 9(5):1705–1711; Milton G *Self-Willed Death or the Bone Pointing Syndrome* June 23 1973 Lancet 1:1435–1436

206. Guyton A, Hall J 1996 *Textbook of Medical Physiology* Sanders, New York p964–965

207. Cohan J *Legally Speaking, Mason v Jacobs* 4Front Magazine April 30 1997

208. Cannon W 1957 *Voodoo Death* Psychosomatic Medicine 19:182–190 (reprinted from American Anthropologist 44:1942); Campinha-Bacote J 1992 *Voodoo Illness* Perspectives in Psychiatric Care 28(1):11–17

209. *The American Medical Association Encyclopedia of Medicine* 1989 Random House, New York p798

210. Reuters News Service report, May 14 1998 on Canadian Amiodarone Myocardial Infarction Arrhythmia Trial (CAMIAT), University of Toronto, Canada

211. Giraldo R 1997 *AIDS and Stressors* Fundacion Arte y Cincia, Medellin; Root-Bernstein R 1993 *Rethinking AIDS* The Free Press, New York; Al Bayati A 1999 *Get All the Facts: HIV Does Not Cause AIDS* Toxi-Health, Dixon, CA

212. Jagge, et al 1983 Annals of Internal Medicine 99:145–151

213. Osterloh J, et al 1984 *Butyl Nitrite Transformation Invitro Anal Toxicology* 8:164–169; Haverkos H, et al 1985 *Disease Manifestation Among Homosexual Men with AIDS* Sexually Transmitted Diseases 12:203–208; Root-Bernstein R 1990 *Do We Know the Cause(s) of AIDS?* Pesp Biol Med 33:480–500

214. Krieger L *Kaposi's Sarcoma, AIDS Link Questioned,* San Francisco Examiner June 5 1992 pA-1,A-17; US Centers for Disease Control *HIV/AIDS Surveillance Report* Year-end reports 1993–1998

215. Marmor, Lancet May 15 1982 (100%); Jaffe, Annals of Internal Medicine 1983 (96%); Harverkos, STD Oct/Nov 1985 (97%); Kaslow, Journal of the American Medical Association 261:23 1989 (96%) Archibald, Epidemiology 3:203 (100%); Duesberg, Genetica, February 1995 (93%)

216. Yardley J, et al 1980 *Immunologic Status in Patients with Giardiasis, Gastroenterology* 78: 421–422; Jaffe, et al 1983 Annals of Internal Medicine 99:145–151

217. Bozzette S, et al 1990 *A Controlled Trial of Early Adjunctive Treatment with Corticosteroids for PCP Pneumonia in AIDS* New England Journal of Medicine 323 (21):145–7; Traltner A, et al 1993 *The Appearance of Kaposi's Sarcoma During Corticosteroid Therapy* Cancer 72 (5):1779–1783

218. Average of two random issues of Edge magazine and Frontiers Gay Biweekly magazine less classified, phone sex, theater and cinema advertisements

219. *Merck Manual* 1992 16th edition p55, Merck Research Laboratories; Glaxo-Wellcome information sheet accompanying Zidovudine

220. Ascher M, et al 1993 *Does Drug Use Cause AIDS?* Nature 362:103–104; Schecter M, et al 1993 *HIV-1 and the Aetiology of AIDS* Lancet 341:658–659; Duesberg P 1993 *Can Epidemiology Determine Whether Drugs or HIV Cause AIDS?* AIDS Forshung 12:627–635

221. Brody, S 1997 *Sex at Risk* Transaction Publishers, New Brunswick; 80%: Potterat et al 1987 JAMA 256 p 12; 65%: Renzullo et al 1990 JAIDS 3, p266–271; 83%–90%: Committee on AIDS Research and the Behavioral, Social, and Statistical Sciences 1989; 69%: Chicago Dept of Public Health, Journal of AIDS 1997; 99.4%: NYC Dept of Health, American Journal of Epidemiology 137:2

222. Duesberg P, Rasnick D 1998 *The AIDS Dilemma: Drug Diseases Based on a Passenger Virus*, Genetica 104: p109 Table 7

Chart References:

1c. Achard G, Bernard H, et al 1909 *Action de la Morphine sur les Proprietes Leucocytaires; Leucodiagnostic du Morphinisme* Bulletin et Memoires de la Societe Medicale des Hopitaux de Paris 28, 3rd Series:958–966; Terry C, Pellens M 1928 *The Opium Problem* Bureau of Social Hygiene of New York; Briggs J, McKerron C, et al 1967 *Severe Systemic Infection Complicating "Mainline" Heroin Addiction* Lancet ii:1227–1231; Sapira J 1968 *The Narcotic Addict as a Medical Patient* Am J Med 45:555–558; Harris P, Garret R 1972 *Susceptibility of Addicts to Infection and Neoplasia* New Engl J Med 287:310; Geller S, Stimmel B 1973 *Diagnostic Confusion from Lymphatic Lesions in Heroin Addicts* Ann Intern Med 78:703–705; Pillari G, Narus J 1973 *Physical Effects of Heroin Addiction* Am J Nursing 73:2105–2109; Brown S, Stimmel B, et al 1974 *Immunologic Dysfunction in Heroin Addicts* Arch Intern Med 134:1001–1006; Louria D 1974 *Infectious Complications of Nonalcoholic Drug Abuse* Annu Rev Med 25:219–231; McDonough R, Madden J, et al 1980 *Alteration of T and Null Lymphocyte Frequencies in the Peripheral Blood of Human Opiate Addicts: In Vivo Evidence of Opiate Receptor Sites on T Lymphocytes* J Immunol 125:2539–2543; Gottlieb M, Schanker H, et al 1981 *Pneumocystis Pneumonia—Los Angeles* Morbidity and Mortality Weekly Reports 30:250–252; Marmor M, Friedman-Kien A, et al 1982 *Risk Factors for Kaposi's Sarcoma in Homosexual Men* Lancet i:1083–1087; Jaffe H, Choi K, et al 1983 *National Case-Control Study of Kaposi's Sarcoma and Pneumocystis Carinii Pneumonia in Homosexual Men: Part 1, Epidemiological Results* Ann Intern Med 99:145–151; Tubaro E, Borelli G, et al 1983 *Effect of Morphine on Resistance to Infection* J Infect Dis 148:656–666; Layon J, Idris A, et al 1984 *Altered T Lymphocyte Subsets in Hospitalized Intravenous Drug Abusers* Arch Intern Med 144:1376–1380; Newell G, Mansell P, et al 1985a *Volatile Nitrites: Use and Adverse Effects Related to the Current Epidemic of Acquired Immune Deficiency Syndrome* Am J Med 78:811–816; Newell G, Mansell P, et al 1985b *Risk Factor Analysis Among Men Referred for Possible Acquired Immune Deficiency Syndrome* Preventive Med 14:81–91; Culver K, Ammann A, et al 1987 *Lymphocyte Abnormalities in Infants Born to Drug-Abusing Mothers* J Pediatr 111:230–235; Donahoe R, Bueso-Ramos C, et al 1987 *Mechanistic Implications of the Findings that Opiates and Other Drugs of Abuse Moderate T-cell Surface Receptors and Antigenic Markers* Ann N.Y. Acad Sci 496:711–721; Bureau of Justice Statistics 1988 *Special Report—Drug Law Violators, 1980–1986* US Department of Justice, Washington DC; Haverkos H, Dougherty J (eds) 1988b *Health Hazards of Nitrite Inhalants* US Department of Health and Human Services, Washington DC; Selwyn P, Feingold A, et al 1988 *Increased Risk of Bacterial Pneumonia in HIV-Infected Intravenous Drug Users without AIDS* AIDS 2:267–272; Novick O, Ochshorn M, et al 1989 *Natural Killer Cell Activity and Lymphocyte Subsets in Parenteral Heroin Abusers and Long-Term Methadone Maintenance Patients* The Journal of Pharmacology and Experimental Therapeutics 250:606–610; Mientjes G, Miedema F, et al 1991 Frequent Injecting Impairs Lymphocyte Reactivity in HIV-Positive and HIV-Negative Drug Users AIDS 5:35–41; Pillai R, Nair B, et al 1991 *AIDS, Drugs of Abuse and the Immune System: A Complex Immunotoxicological Network* Arch Toxicol 65:609–617; Larrat P, Zierler S 1993 *Entangled Epidemics: Cocaine Use and HIV Disease* J Psychoactive Drugs 25:207–221; Mientjes G, van Ameijden E, et al 1993 *Clinical Symptoms Associated with Seroconversion for HIV-1 among Misusers of Intravenous Drugs: Comparison with Homosexual Seroconverters and Infected and Non-Infected Intravenous Drug Misusers* Br. Med. J. 306:371–373; Sadownick D 1994 *Kneeling at the Crystal Cathedral* Genre December/January 1994 p40–45, 86–90; Ratajczak H, Thomas P, et al 1995 Local Versus Systemic Immunotoxicity of Isobutyl Nitrite Following Subchronic Inhalation Exposure of Female B6C3F1 Mice Fundamental and Applied Technology 27:177–184; Brettle R 1996 *Clinical Features of Drug Use and Drug Use Related to HIV* Int J STD & AIDS 7:151–165

2c. Jaffe H, Choi K, et al 1983 *National Case-Control Study of Kaposi's Sarcoma and Pneumocystis Carinii Pneumonia in Homosexual Men: Part 1, Epidemiological Results* Ann Intern Med 99:145–151; Newell G, Adamas S, et al 1984 *Toxicity, Immunosuppressive Effects and Carcinogenic Potential of Volatile Nitrites: Possible Relationship to Kaposi's Sarcoma* Pharmacotherapy 4:284–291; Haverkos H, Pinsky P, et al 1985 *Disease Manifestation Among Homosexual Men with Acquired Immunodeficiency Syndrome: A Possible Role of Nitrites in Kaposi's Sarcoma* J Sex Trans Dis 12:203–208; Haverkos H, *Kaposi's Sarcoma and Nitrite Inhalants* In: Psychological, Neuropsychiatric and Substance Abuse Aspects of AIDS by Bridge T, Heather H, Johnson M (eds) Raven Press, New York p165–172; Haverkos H, Dougherty J 1988a *Health Hazards of Nitrite Inhalants* Am J Med 84:479–482; Archer C, Spittle M, et al 1989 *Kaposi's Sarcoma in a Homosexual—10 Years On* Clin Exper Dermatol 14:233–236; Friedman-Kien A, Saltzman B, et al 1990 *Kaposi's Sarcoma in HIV-Negative Homosexual Men* Lancet 335:168–169; Marquart K, Engst R, et al 1991 *An 8-Year History of Kaposi's Sarcoma in an HIV-Negative Bisexual Man* AIDS 5:346–348; Safai B, Peralta H, et al 1991 *Kaposi's Sarcoma among HIV-Negative High Risk Populations* VII International Conference on AIDS, Florence, Italy

3c. Pillari G, Narus J 1973 *Physical Effects of Heroin Addiction* Am J Nursing 73:2105–2109; Stoneburner R, Des Jarlais D, et al 1988 *A Larger Spectrum of Severe HIV-1-Related Disease in Intravenous Drug Users in New York City* Science 242:916–919; Rogers M, Ou C, et al 1989 *Use of the Polymerase Chain Reaction for Early Detection of the Proviral Sequences of Human Immunodeficiency Virus in Infants Born to Seropositive Mothers* N Engl J Med 320:1649–1654

4c. Gottlieb M, Schanker H, et al 1981 *Pneumocystis Pneumonia—Los Angeles* Morbidity and Mortality Weekly Reports 30:250–252; Jaffe H, Choi K, et al 1983 *National Case-Control Study of Kaposi's Sarcoma and Pneumocystis Carinii Pneumonia in Homosexual Men: Part 1, Epidemiological Results* Ann Intern Med 99:145–151; Mathur-Wagh U, Enlow R, et al 1984 *Longitudinal Study of Persistent Generalized Lymphadenopathy in Homosexual Men: Relation to Acquired Immunodeficiency Syndrome* Lancet i:1033–1038; Mathur-Wagh U, Mildvan D, et al 1985 *Follow-Up of 4½ Years on Homosexual Men with Generalized Lymphadenopathy* N Engl J Med 313:1542–1543; Selwyn P, Feingold A, et al 1988 *Increased Risk of Bacterial Pneumonia in HIV-Infected Intravenous Drug Users without AIDS* AIDS 2:267–272; Stoneburner R, Des Jarlais D, et al 1988 *A Larger Spectrum of Severe HIV-1-Related Disease in Intravenous Drug Users in New York City* Science 242:916–919; Ettinger N, Albin R 1989 *A Review of the Respiratory Effects of Smoking Cocaine* Am J Med 87:664–668; Mientjes G, van Ameijden E, et al 1993 *Clinical Symptoms Associated with Seroconversion for HIV-1 among Misusers of Intravenous Drugs: Comparison with Homosexual Seroconverters and Infected and Non-Infected Intravenous Drug Misusers* Br. Med. J. 306:371–373; Hayes T, Altman R, et al 1994 *HIV-Related Deaths from Selected Infectious Diseases among Persons without AIDS in New Jersey* Journal of Acquired Immune Deficiency Syndromes 7:1074–1078; Brettle R 1996 *Clinical Features of Drug Use and Drug Use Related to HIV* Int J STD & AIDS 7:151–165

5c. Geller S, Stimmel B 1973 *Diagnostic Confusion from Lymphatic Lesions in Heroin Addicts* Ann Intern Med 78:703–705; Pillari G, Narus J 1973 *Physical Effects of Heroin Addiction* Am J Nursing 73:2105–2109; Espinoza P, Bouchard I, et al 1987 *High Prevalence of Infection by Hepatitis B Virus and HIV in Incarcerated French Drug Addicts* Gastroenterologie Clinique et Biologique 11:288–292; Des Jarlais D, Friedman S, et al 1988 *Risk Reduction of the Acquired Immune Deficiency Syndrome among Intravenous Drug Users* In: AIDS and IV Drug Abusers: Current Perspectives by Galea R, Lewis B, Baker L (eds) National Health Publishing, Owings Mills, MD p97–109; Brettle R 1996 *Clinical Features of Drug Use and Drug Use Related to HIV* Int J STD & AIDS 7:151–165

6c. Firooznia H, Seliger G, et al 1973 *Disseminated Extrapulmonary Tuberculosis in Association with Heroin Addiction* Radiology 109:291–296; Courtwright D 1982 *Dark Paradise: Opiate Addiction in America Before 1940* Harvard University Press, Cambridge, MA; Layon J, Idris A, et al 1984 *Altered T Lymphocyte Subsets in Hospitalized Intravenous Drug Abusers* Arch Intern Med 144:1376–1380; Stoneburner R, Des Jarlais D, et al 1988 *A Larger Spectrum of Severe HIV-1-Related Disease in Intravenous Drug Users in New York City* Science 242:916–919; Braun M, Truman B, et al 1989 *Increasing Incidence of Tuberculosis in a Prison Inmate Population, Associated with HIV Infection* J Am Med Assoc 261:393–397; Brudney K, Dobkin J 1991 *Resurgent Tuberculosis in New York City* Am Rev Respir Dis 144:744–749; Hayes T, Altman R, et al 1994 *HIV-Related Deaths from Selected Infectious Diseases among Persons without AIDS in New Jersey* Journal of Acquired Immune Deficiency Syndromes 7:1074–1078

7c. Pillari G, Narus J 1973 *Physical Effects of Heroin Addiction* Am J Nursing 73:2105–2109; Des Jarlais D, Friedman S, et al1988 *Risk Reduction of the Acquired Immune Deficiency Syndrome among Intravenous Drug Users* In: AIDS and IV Drug Abusers: Current Perspectives by Galea R, Lewis B, Baker L (eds) National Health Publishing, Owings Mills, MD p97–109; Brettle R 1996 *Clinical Features of Drug Use and Drug Use Related to HIV* Int J STD & AIDS 7:151–165; Bergling T 1997 *All Methed Up: Doing Crystal Meth Will Lift You Up Until You Break* Genre 53:October p45–47,88; McEvoy A, Kitchen N, et al 1998 *Intracerebral Haemorrhage Caused by Drug Abuse* Lancet 351:1029

8c. Stoneburner R, Des Jarlais D, et al 1988 *A Larger Spectrum of Severe HIV-1-Related Disease in Intravenous Drug Users in New York City* Science 242:916–919; Koch T July 30 1990 *Uninfected Children of HIV-Infected Mothers May Still Suffer Nervous Problems* CDC AIDS Weekly p9; Aylward E, Butz A, et al 1992 *Cognitive and Motor Development in Infants at Risk for Human Immunodeficiency Virus* Am J Dis Child 146:218–222; Larrat P, Zierler S 1993 *Entangled Epidemics: Cocaine Use and HIV Disease* J Psychoactive Drugs 25:207–221; Hayes T, Altman R, et al 1994 *HIV-Related Deaths from Selected Infectious Diseases among Persons without AIDS in New Jersey* Journal of Acquired Immune Deficiency Syndromes 7:1074–1078; Brettle R 1996 *Clinical Features of Drug Use and Drug Use Related to HIV* Int J STD & AIDS 7:151–165; McEvoy A, Kitchen N, et al 1998 *Intracerebral Haemorrhage Caused by Drug Abuse* Lancet 351:1029

9c. Des Jarlais D, Friedman S, et al 1988 *Risk Reduction of the Acquired Immune Deficiency Syndrome among Intravenous Drug Users* In: AIDS and IV Drug Abusers: Current Perspectives by Galea R, Lewis B, Baker L (eds) National Health Publishing, Owings Mills, MD p97–109; Muñoz A, Vlahov D, et al 1992 *Prognostic Indicators for Development of AIDS among Intravenous Drug Users* J Acquir Immune Defic Syndr 5:694–700; Brettle R 1996 *Clinical Features of Drug Use and Drug Use Related to HIV* Int J STD & AIDS 7:151–165

10c. Des Jarlais D, Friedman S, et al 1988 *Risk Reduction of the Acquired Immune Deficiency Syndrome among Intravenous Drug Users* In: AIDS and IV Drug Abusers: Current Perspectives by Galea R, Lewis B, Baker L (eds) National Health Publishing, Owings Mills, MD p97–109; Ettinger N, Albin R 1989 *A Review of the Respiratory Effects of Smoking Cocaine* Am J Med 87:664–668; Brettle R 1996 *Clinical Features of Drug Use and Drug Use Related to HIV* Int J STD & AIDS 7:151–165

11c. Savona S, Nardi M, et al 1985 *Thrombocytopenic Purpura in Narcotics Addicts* Ann Intern Med 102:737–741

12c. Fricker H, Segal S 1978 *Narcotic Addiction, Pregnancy, and the Newborn* Am J Dis Child 132:360–366; Lifschitz M, Wilson G, et al 1983 *Fetal and Postnatal growth of Children Born to Narcotic-Dependent Women* J Pediatr 102:686–691; Alroomi L, Davidson J, et al 1988 *Maternal Narcotic Abuse and the Newborn* Arch Dis Child 63:81–83; Rogers M, Ou C, et al 1989 *Use of the Polymerase Chain Reaction for Early Detection of the Proviral Sequences of Human Immunodeficiency Virus in Infants Born to Seropositive Mothers* N Engl J Med 320:1649–1654; Toufexis A May 13 1991 *Innocent Victims* Time p56–60; Finnegan L, Mellot J, et al 1992 *Perinatal Exposure to Cocaine: Human Studies* In: Cocaine: Pharmacology, Physiology and Clinical Strategies by Lakoski J, Galloway M, White F (eds) CRC Press, Boca Raton, FL p391–409; Larrat P, Zierler S 1993 *Entangled Epidemics: Cocaine Use and HIV Disease* J Psychoactive Drugs 25:207–221

13c. Des Jarlais D, Friedman S, et al 1988 *Risk Reduction of the Acquired Immune Deficiency Syndrome among Intravenous Drug Users* In: AIDS and IV Drug Abusers: Current Perspectives by Galea R, Lewis B, Baker L (eds) National Health Publishing, Owings Mills, MD p97–109; Brettle R 1996 *Clinical Features of Drug Use and Drug Use Related to HIV* Int J STD & AIDS 7:151–165

14c. Larrat P, Zierler S 1993 *Entangled Epidemics: Cocaine Use and HIV Disease* J Psychoactive Drugs 25:207–221; Brettle R 1996 *Clinical Features of Drug Use and Drug Use Related to HIV* Int J STD & AIDS 7:151–165

15c. Wilson J, Kalasinsky K, et al 1996 *Striatal Dopamine Nerve Terminal Markers in Human, Chronic Methamphetamine Users* Nature Medicine 2:699–703

16c. Pillari G, Narus J 1973 *Physical Effects of Heroin Addiction* Am J Nursing 73:2105–2109

17c. Pillari G, Narus J 1973 *Physical Effects of Heroin Addiction* Am J Nursing 73:2105–2109; Brettle R 1996 *Clinical Features of Drug Use and Drug Use Related to HIV* Int J STD & AIDS 7:151–165

18c. Dismukes W, Karchmer A, et al 1968 *Viral Hepatitis Associated with Illicit Parenteral Use of Drugs* J Am Med Assoc 206:1048–1052; Pillari G, Narus J 1973 *Physical Effects of Heroin Addiction* Am J Nursing 73:2105–2109; Layon J, Idris A, et al 1984 *Altered T Lymphocyte Subsets in Hospitalized Intravenous Drug Abusers* Arch Intern Med 144:1376–1380

19c. Brettle R 1996 *Clinical Features of Drug Use and Drug Use Related to HIV* Int J STD & AIDS 7:151–165

20c. Layon J, Idris A, et al 1984 *Altered T Lymphocyte Subsets in Hospitalized Intravenous Drug Abusers* Arch Intern Med 144:1376–1380; Stoneburner R, Des Jarlais D, et al 1988 *A Larger Spectrum of Severe HIV-1-Related Disease in Intravenous Drug Users in New York City* Science 242:916–919; Mientjes G, van Ameijden E, et al 1993 *Clinical Symptoms Associated with Seroconversion for HIV-1 among Misusers of Intravenous Drugs: Comparison with Homosexual Seroconverters and Infected and Non-Infected Intravenous Drug Misusers* Br. Med. J. 306:371–373; Brettle R 1996 *Clinical Features of Drug Use and Drug Use Related to HIV* Int J STD & AIDS 7:151–165

223. Indiana Hemophilia Foundation. Source: Duesberg P 1996 *Inventing the AIDS Virus* Regnery Publishing, Washington DC p287–288

224. *Blood Transfusions: Fewer Blood Transfusions Save Lives* United Press International February 10 1999; Hebert P, et al New England Journal of Medicine February 11 1999

225. Brody, S 1997 *Sex at Risk* Transaction Publishers, New Brunswick; 80%: Potterat et al 1987 JAMA 256 p 12; 65%: Renzullo, et al 1990 JAIDS 3, p266–271; 83%–90%: Committee on AIDS Research and the Behavioral, Social, and Statistical Sciences 1989; 69%: Chicago Dept of Public Health, Journal of AIDS 1997; 99.4%: NYC Dept of Health, American Journal of Epidemiology 137:2

226. Fumento M Washington Times June 8 1999

227. US Centers for Disease Control 1999 *HIV/AIDS Surveillance Report* Year-end 1998 p14 Table 5

228. Altman L *Outside of US and Europe HIV Transmission is Through Heterosexual Contact* New York Times November 2 1993

229. Biggar R, et al 1985 *ELISA HTLV Retrovirus Antibody Reactivity Associated With Malaria* Lancet ii 520–543; Charmot G, Simon F 1990 *HIV Infection and Malaria* Revue Du Practien 40:2124; Bush, et al Journal of AIDS 5:872 1992; Kashala O, et al 1994 *Infection with HIV-1 and Human T Cell Lymhotropic Viruses Among Leprosy Patients and Contacts* Journal of Infectious Diseases 169:292–304

230. Piatak M, et al 1993 Science 259:1749–53

231. World Health Organization annual conversions rates. Source: Willner R *Deadly Deception* Peltec Publishing p39–41

232. Benthen B, et al *Insights from the Tricontinental Seroconverter Study* AIDS June 18 1998 12:1039–1045; New England Journal of Medicine 1995 332:209; Journal of Infectious Diseases 1996 173:60

233. Buchbinder S, et al 1994 *Long Term HIV 1 Infection Without Immunologic Progression* AIDS 8:1123; Pantaleo G, et al 1995 *Studies in Subjects with Long-Term Non-Progressive HIV Infection* New England Journal of Medicine 332(4):209–216; Muñoz A, et al 1995 *Long-Term Survivors of HIV-1 Infection* Journal of AIDS and Human Retrovirology April 15 8(5):496–505

234. Journal InterAM Medical Health Association 1992 1:1–8

235. Callen M *Surviving AIDS* Harper-Collins Publishing; Root-Bernstein R *Rethinking AIDS* The Free Press, New York p361–363; Time Magazine March 22 1993; Gregory S, Leonardo B 1992 *They Conquered AIDS: True Life Adventures*; MacIntyre R, *Mortal Men: Living with Asymptomatic HIV* University Press, Rutgers; Chaitow L, Strohecker J 1997 *You Don't Have to Die: Unraveling the AIDS Myth* Future Medicine Publishing

236. Genetica 1996 *AIDS: Virus or Drug Induced?* p3–22; Ostrom N *The T4 Myth* New York Native May 2 1994

237. Bird A 1996 *Non-HIV AIDS* Journal of Antimicrobial Chemotherapy 37(B):171–183; Haynes S *California State Department of Health Services AIDS Study*. Source: Farber C SPIN magazine May 1994

238. Mosley J *Transfusion Safety Study Group Report* presented at 1993 International AIDS conference. Source: Farber C SPIN magazine May 1994

239. Fleming T, De Mets D *Surrogate End Points in Clinical Trials: Are We Being Misled?* Annals of Internal Medicine October 1 1996 125:605–613

240. Carney W, Rubin R, et al *Analysis of T Lymphocyte Subsets in CMV Mononucleosis* June 1981 Journal of Immunology; Feeney C, Bryzman S, et al October 1995 *T-Lymphocyte Subsets in Acute Illness* Critical Care Medicine 23 (10):1680–1685

241. US Centers for Disease Control, 1998 *Guidelines for the Use of Antiretroviral Agents in HIV-Infected Adults and Adolescents*

242. Source for entire section: The American Association of Oriental Medicine *Understanding Oriental Medicine, Acupuncture and Herbology* Catasauqua, PA; Cassileth B PhD *The Alternative Medicine Handbook* WW Norton & Co, New York; *The Complete Guide to Alternative And Conventional Treatments* Time Life Books, Alexandria; Mortimore D *The Complete Illustrated Guide to Nutritional Healing*, Element Press, Boston; *New Choices in Natural Healing*, Rodale Press Inc., Emmaus; Tips J PhD *Your Liver...Your Lifeline: Detoxification and Rejuvenation for the Whole Body* Apple-A-Day Press, Austin; Jensen B PhD DC *Tissue Cleansing Through Bowel Management* Bernard Jensen International, Escondido

243. POZ Magazine July 1992

244. Schwartz D, et al 1997 *Extensive Evaluation of a Seronegative Participant in an HIV-1 Vaccine Trial as a Result of False-Positive PCR*, Lancet Vol 350 No 9073 p256

245. Wall Street Journal May 1 1996

246. *American Heritage Dictionary Second College Edition* Houghton Mittlin Company, Boston p492

247. Documentary film *HIV=AIDS: Fact or Fraud* Starvision Productions Denver CO 1997; CNN Website *Massive Trial of AIDS Vaccine to Begin in Thailand* February 10 1999 8:27 pm EST

248. Altman L *Inherited Factor May Play Role in Risk of AIDS* New York Times May 10 1987

Appendix: The Other Side of AIDS

It is commonly believed that people who test HIV positive are infected with an incurable virus, and that without daily doses of multiple medicines, the virus will replicate unchecked and lead to an inevitable series of illnesses and infections that invariably result in death.

As AIDS research has replaced the hope for a cure with the goal of creating more powerful anti-HIV treatments, AIDS organizations have directed their efforts to promoting and supplying drugs, while public health officials push for widespread and even mandatory testing to identify those in need of treatment.

Treatment=Life, the newest battle cry in the war on AIDS, is regarded by most as an absolute truth, a rule without exception. While the media makes occasional mention of an HIV positive who lives without the drugs, such people are regarded as few in number, and usually described as mysteriously and temporarily lucky.

This narrow view of AIDS leaves the general public unaware of the fact that there are thousands of men, women and children throughout the world who are naturally well many years after testing HIV positive. Of all the unanswered questions about AIDS, perhaps the most compelling one is why healthy people whose lives defy the HIV=AIDS=Death paradigm are being ignored. The following are just a few of the voices that need to be heard if we are ever to understand and resolve AIDS.*

> "I tested positive for HIV over Memorial Day weekend 1986. I believe I was infected two years prior to that, so I have been 'living with HIV' for at least 15 years. Four years ago, a.k.a. the ninth year of my death sentence, I finally allowed myself to recognize an undeniable fact of my own life. Without any medical intervention, including 'antiretroviral' medication, I was neither a) sick nor b) dead.

> "My path has taken me from a firm belief that HIV causes AIDS, to believing the immune system could be enhanced with nontoxic alternatives to antiretrovirals, to questioning whether HIV causes AIDS. This progression in thinking about HIV/AIDS is a direct result of my own personal experience. I understand that the notion that HIV might not cause AIDS is upsetting for many. I'm not raising the question merely to be provocative. The possibility that a horrendous mistake has been made is disturbing to me.

> "What's really ironic is that my story is a positive one though I'm almost ashamed to admit it. Is it the last taboo: discussing your non-death from AIDS? But I can't resist—I have to say it. These past four years, once I learned to let go of the fear, have been the most positive, life-affirming years of my life.

---

* Contact information for each person who provided a testimonial including their complete name, address and phone number may be made available to individuals or organizations upon request.

"As they say at Alive & Well: 'Relax, it's only information.' There is another side to the HIV/AIDS story. I think everybody with HIV or AIDS should be allowed to hear about it and make an informed decision for him or herself. A little free speech, open debate, and civil discourse never hurt anybody. To all doubters, I say take a deep breath, open your mind, and read."

David Fink, San Francisco, CA

"In 1985, at the age of 25, having heard so much about the 'AIDS epidemic,' I decided to take the test. I tested positive. I went for a second opinion and again the result was positive. Since I had heard and read that the virus could be dormant for a long time, I opted to eat well, exercise, take high quality vitamins and limit 'risky sex.' However, my gut feeling was that something wasn't adding up with AIDS, and I almost immediately chose not to accept the virus as a detriment to my health.

"Throughout the years I've lived my life almost as if AIDS didn't exist but still gathered information from various sources. I seldom take prescription drugs and never get flu shots. I seldom see a general practitioner and see a homeopath for little things that come up once in a while. I've had shingles three times due to job stress but bounce back quite rapidly. I don't even take aspirin since I almost never get headaches. To this day, I have never been hospitalized and have not taken any of the drugs that are supposed to control or eradicate HIV."

Cirilo Juarez, Los Angeles, CA

"When I tested positive in 1988, I was told I had only three years to live. Twelve years later, I'm doing just fine. I have never taken any AIDS drugs even though they were suggested and even pushed.

"For so many years, my HIV status was a secret I kept to myself. I only told people on a need-to-know basis and that was always hell to do. HIV disrupted my life and my relationships on many levels. When I found out that there were facts about HIV and AIDS I hadn't been told, it changed my life. I'm more open now, I help other people get educated about their choices.

"In 1996 I got married—five years after I was supposed to be dead! I'm very alive and healthy and wish people would listen to me and other people like me for a change. Fear and isolation is what really kills people who test HIV positive. I fully believe that the HIV=AIDS hypothesis is a violation of our rights to life and liberty, and that ignorance is the real epidemic."

Michele M, Monterey, CA

"I've known over 200 people who died of so-called AIDS. Every one of them had sufficient drug abuse or medical terrorism to account for their immune suppression. When I was told on January 7, 1988 that I was

HIV positive and had about two years to live, it came as a complete shock to me because I did not have a history of what was considered high-risk behavior.

"What came as a bigger shock than testing positive was learning that no one was interested in investigating any natural cures. What it boiled down to was, if it wasn't a drug, they didn't want to know about it. By 1992 I had learned enough to convince me that AIDS was the greatest medical error of all time.

"As I write this it has been eleven years since I first got tested. I've never developed any AIDS-defining illnesses. In fact, I haven't had a cold in 19 years. I ride a bicycle for transportation all year round. I take no medications, no medical treatments, no vitamins or herbal supplements—just good food and ten minutes a day of exercise for the immune system.

"Had I listened to the doctors in 1988, I wouldn't be here today. Now in my mid-fifties, I have a better body than I've ever had in my life. Most of my friends are close to half my age. HIV cost me a lot. I lost my income, my savings and a lot of friends. I thank God that I was smart enough to 'just say no' to the doctors, so it didn't cost me my health. If anything, as a result of what I learned, I'm healthier today than I've ever been."

Ed Lieb, New York, NY

"I took an HIV test in May of 1990. It was recommended that I do so because I was pregnant. Since I come from a small town and have had only long-term relationships and remain in touch with my former boyfriends, I didn't even consider the possibility of testing anything but negative. I know all of them and they are all fine. Instead, the test came back inconclusive.

"I took it again and that one gave a positive result. I was told that the change from inconclusive to positive meant that I had a new infection. Even though that made no sense as far as the circumstances of my life, I believed it.

"The positive result left me in total shock. I believed everything I was told at the time including that I would become sick and die within five years. Since my T cells were high, I was not instructed to take any medicines. If they had been lower, or if they pushed me like they do to people today, I think I would be dead by now.

"I was told that I would have to decide what to do about my baby. The information I was given left me without much choice. They said that there were two scenarios: I could live long enough to watch my baby die of AIDS or I could leave my baby without a mother when I died of AIDS, knowing that my baby would die soon after me. How could I even think of having a child in such circumstances? Believing in the death sentence I had been given, I agreed to have a second trimester abortion. It was a terrible, terrible experience and the decision haunts me to this day. Knowing what I know now, I feel like the baby was killed because of the bad information I was given.

"About two years later I met a man and we became involved in a four-year relationship. He was absolutely certain that HIV did not cause AIDS. He had done a lot of research on the whole thing and decided that being HIV positive didn't mean anything. You would think I would have been happy to be in a relationship with a man who was convinced I would be all right. Instead, I was miserable. I worried about him constantly. I was frustrated that he wouldn't take my 'condition' seriously. I was also angry and bitter about having to die of AIDS. At that time, according to the doctors, I was in my last year of life. I still believed this even though I wasn't ill. We ended up breaking up because I was so bitter, sad and angry. I was all caught up in the idea that I was going to die.

"In 1996, I found Alive & Well Alternatives and finally read the information. It has given me the facts and the strength to realize I am not dying and has totally changed my world. I've never been on any AIDS medicines and I would never take them knowing what I know now. I am still sorry for the baby I didn't have, but am glad to be alive and to know that I can stay healthy."

Iola Marin, Los Angeles, CA

"I tested positive in 1989 and have been living in wellness without the meds for ten years, something that still shocks people even though I've always been just fine. After watching my friends on AIDS drug therapies get sick and die, I decided that HIV drugs are poison and you can't poison yourself back to health. I learned to do nothing 'for HIV.' Instead, I focus on being healthy."

Kim Freitas, Los Angeles, CA

"In 1989, my husband Philip was diagnosed HIV positive during qualification for life insurance. We immediately saw a specialist who gave him six months to live. To add to our nightmare, I also tested HIV positive. We couldn't believe that two people like us, nice people from nice families, were having to deal firsthand with AIDS.

"We went to an internationally renowned doctor at the forefront of AIDS research who confirmed Philip's prognosis. Even though we were frightened and upset, we felt fortunate to be in the care of a respected leader on the cutting edge of AIDS developments. This doctor provided Philip with experimental drugs six months to a year before they were available to the public. At least 10 times, the doctor told me that Philip would not pull through whatever infection he was going through. Ten times, I went through the fear, heartache, and panic that I was losing my husband. Six years after being told he had just months to live, Philip died in my arms. I know that the five years he added to his life were generated by his deep faith, his passion for life, and his love for me.

"I had been positive and healthy for seven years when the doctor decided, due to a drop in my T cells, that it was time for me to start the medicines. Until then, I had never questioned my doctor, the drugs, or the idea that

HIV causes AIDS. I lived in fear of getting sick although I was never ill during the entire seven years. Once I was told it was my turn to take the drugs, I realized I had to make the most important decision of my life.

"My doctor gave me no facts or education about the drug treatments, only emotionally charged orders and fear. I had seen what the drugs did to my husband and I was terrified. In desperation, I called Christine Maggiore. We had met in 1992 in a support group for HIV positive women. Even though I liked and respected her, I questioned the choices she had made to reject not only the AIDS drugs, but the whole idea that HIV causes AIDS. What she said didn't just rock the boat, it sunk it. I was frustrated that my life was on the line and the only person I could turn to for help was Christine. I had no one to confer or consult with. My husband was gone and I couldn't call my family—all highly successful professionals—and ask them to help me evaluate information from some lady with a website and flyers.

"I asked Christine to give me just the scientific information and nothing else. No stories or emotional hype, only the facts. I had to go to her office several times to read because I became so distraught that I couldn't continue for more than 15 minutes. Everything I read described and explained what I had been through with my husband. My worst fears were being confirmed—the drugs had made my husband suffer tremendously, and had eventually killed him. And until that day, I hadn't been able to hear what Christine had tried to tell me.

"I started attending Alive & Well events to learn more. HIV positives who chose not to follow mainstream medicine encouraged me to think for myself. I felt like I was on a dangerous, courageous and mind-expanding journey. Ultimately I decided that the AIDS drugs were not for me. I decided to trust my own life.

"After I made the decision, I took my last diagnostic test, a viral load for a study I have since dropped. A year before I did this, I had already decided AIDS was no longer a part of my life; I had declared myself 'AIDS-free.' I find my 'undetectable' result an affirmation of this decision. I currently see a doctor of naturopathic medicine who helps me attain my health goals. I have safely lost 65 pounds and look and feel better than I have in many years.

"When we believe the doctors and accept that we are going to die, this belief, inconspicuous at first, must eventually manifest in our lives. Believing in health is the first step to creating a healthy life. Holding the possibility of health is everything."

Cynthia Rogers, Los Angeles, CA

"I tested positive in 1990, and ten years later I am healthy and medication-free. When I was first told I was positive I went through the standard terror with my life flashing before my eyes. I followed my doctors orders for treatment with AZT and soon after I became ill. I had flu-like symptoms day and night. It got to the point where I'd come home from work and just collapse on the couch. When I told my doctor how I felt he said 'Well, what do you expect, you're HIV positive!?'

"After a year of feeling sick, I listened to my inner voice and quit AZT. Except for a brief foray into ddI, I've been off meds ever since. I have three recommendations for anyone who tests positive—education, education, education about all aspects and points of view on HIV and AIDS. And remember, people do get sick sometimes, so if it happens, be realistic and don't freak out. Don't automatically assume it's related to HIV. My doctor now classifies me as a 'long-term non-progressor!'"

Erik Dahlgren, Los Angeles, CA

"It all started in the winter of 1984 with swollen glands, a rash on my legs, and night sweats. I saw a doctor who took my temperature, said I had a slight fever, felt the swollen glands and kidded 'you aren't gay, are you?' When I said that I was, his tone immediately changed. He went out of the examination room and I heard him ask his nurse to take my blood. He said this could be AIDS so be sure and use gloves. Her response was an emphatic no. The doctor came back in the room wearing a surgical mask and gloves. After many pathetic attempts to find a vein he finally got a few vials.

"Three days later he called and said the blood results were not good. This was before the Western Blot and ELISA were available. He said that my T cell count was below 200 and it appeared that I had AIDS. He told me that he thought I would be dead within six months, and it would not be pretty.

"I saw another doctor for a second opinion and his conclusions were the same. My T cells were shot and opportunistic infection would set in any day. I started taking an experimental drug I smuggled in from Mexico but the doctor didn't want to follow up with me to see if it was doing any good. He just told me to take two pills four times a day, and when I asked for how long, he said 'forever.'

"I didn't feel any worse and continued to go weekly for blood work and was always told my counts were terrible. This continued for two months until the lab technician demanded payment. I told her my HMO covered it but she said 'They aren't paying for this, you need to pay today.' I took off the rubber tube she was using to constrict my vein, walked out and never went back. I continued with the experimental drug for about a year, until the FDA decided that it was basically worthless. My spirits dropped dramatically but something was funny, I was still alive.

"Each day after work I would go home, eat dinner, look for Kaposi's Sarcoma and thrush, feel how swollen my glands were, go to bed and wait to die. I slept 20 hours a day on the weekends. I remember I took a vacation to Mexico and spent it in bed. The news was full of AIDS articles and they always ended with 'no one has ever recovered' or 'everyone with this disease dies.'

"My symptoms, except the swollen glands, all went away after about eight months. I made it a point never to go back to my HMO doctors. If I had a sinus infection or any other medical problem, I went to one of the urgent care centers and always paid cash.

"Then AZT came onto the scene. I think it was a television news conference with Dr. Gallo saying what a remarkable discovery it was. I didn't trust the man, there was something wrong. I never pursued it and kept to my regimen of working, eating, sleeping and waiting for the disease to take me. By then, several of my friends had been diagnosed with AIDS, all were put on AZT, and all died within one year. Each of their doctors had understated the side effects and exaggerated the curative aspects of this drug.

"In 1997, I made an appointment with an HMO doctor for a problem unrelated to HIV or AIDS. He said something that startled me: 'You know, we have made quite a bit of progress with AIDS and there are many new drugs you might consider.' I said I had no symptoms and didn't think that was for me. He said 'You need to start them before you have the symptoms.' I laughed to myself and told him I would think about it. In 1999, 15 years after I was given six months to live, I celebrated my 47th birthday."

Don McCoy, Laguna Beach, CA

"While living in New York City in 1982, my doctor informed me that I had contracted 'the virus that's affecting gay men.' Remember GRID? I was later diagnosed HIV positive as soon as the current testing methods became available.

"Fast-forward 18 years. I run a successful interior design business, I work out several times a week, I enjoy hiking and practicing T'ai Chi. In all this time I have never had any opportunistic infections. I enjoy good health, not so much for what I am doing with my life but rather for what I am not doing: I am not taking toxic HIV-related pharmaceutical drugs. It's the drugs, not the virus, that are killing people who test positive! I congratulate myself for having the courage to open my mind and I thank groups like Alive & Well for providing me with life-affirming information."

Michael Koslosky, Los Angeles, CA

"I am 28 years old and approaching a healthy 29, an age a doctor once told me I would never reach. When I was 20, I moved from Australia to Japan where I spent a year as an entertainer singing on a cruise ship and in various bars and restaurants in Osaka. Toward the end of my stay, me and my partner Ruichi and a group of friends visited the historic city of Kyoto. While we were there, we all went to an HIV testing clinic. I had been having frequent unprotected sex with Ruichi for about three months, and prior to that I had unprotected sex with one of the other guys getting tested, so it seemed that I should join them and take the test.

"At the time, my primary source of HIV and AIDS information, like the majority of the general public, was the media. I remember one TV commercial that aired in Australia that portrayed AIDS as the Grim Reaper in a bowling alley. He used his deadly balls to knock out men, women and children who appeared as helpless bowling pins.

"Our test results arrived by mail two weeks later, all in the same envelope, and we opened it together. The results were in Japanese so Ruichi read them out loud going down the list one by one. 'Riuchi: negative,' he looked at me and smiled. 'David: negative, Renee: negative, Dean...' and he paused, eyes wide. My heart skipped a beat as I waited for him to continue: 'Dean: positive.'

"My first reaction was disbelief. I was healthy and so was everyone I had ever slept with. I figured I was going to die, and knowing so little about AIDS, I figured I had three to six months left before I would be bowled over. I was so ashamed. I called all my past sex partners advising them to be tested. All of them were negative.

"I went into a phase of denial. I convinced myself that my test result was wrong. I waited three months and then tested again in Australia. The sympathy I received at the testing clinic was not encouraging. The most optimistic doctor gave me 10 years to live but noted that at least two of those years would include devastating disease. This beat my own prognosis of six months, but did not give me much to look forward to.

"After a few months of soul searching, the existence of the mind-body connection occurred to me. I quickly discovered I was not the only one to recognize that disease was more than a random physical mishap. Since then, and for more than seven years, I have read everything I can find on alternative medicine, science, self-help and spirituality. I've also tried many alternative therapies and techniques for improving the mind and the body. I have never taken any medication, but have instead focused on maintaining health. I've learned to keep an open mind to new ideas, and not to believe everything experts have to say.

"I no longer believe that HIV causes AIDS, and this belief is not denial. I experienced denial when I suppressed my fears of dying. My belief may not be proved by government-funded AIDS research, but the government has done little that would suggest it cares about the well-being of humanity above all else. Avoiding death is not my number one priority—living is.

"What I find hardest is living with the stigma of HIV. I'm young, healthy, intelligent and very well-educated on HIV and AIDS, yet I am isolated by the fear and ignorance surrounding a condition I don't even believe in. Being a leader rather than a follower can be lonely and difficult. Maintaining a stance against the majority of the human population is a trying task. I don't have the time to educate everyone, even if they were interested, and when I do tell others about what I know, they are so convinced that HIV=AIDS=Death that they think I'm doomed and that my optimism is merely fear or hope or both.

"I do have hope. I hope that people will look deeper and listen more. That they will demand to be treated as precious beings more important than politics, money, and abstract theory. It takes people like us to be the first and the most determined. Life goes on, chose to be a part of it!"

Dean W, Los Angeles, CA

"I tested positive in May of 1995. That may not seem terribly interesting until you consider that prior to the test, I had never had 'unprotected sex.' After extensive research I decided that the AIDS meds were not for me. I found out about Alive & Well through my acupuncturist.

"I am happy to say that I am just as healthy as I was when I was in high school, except for my usual allergies and chronic flat feet. While I am not technically a 'long-term survivor,' I am here to encourage you to do what I did: research for yourself, get the information and make up your own mind."

Lou Rosenblate, Hollywood, CA

"I was required by law to take an HIV test in June of 1995. The test is mandatory in Colorado for pregnant women, and I was expecting my second child. I was shocked when the results came back positive because I'd been married and monogamous for nine years. My situation became even more incomprehensible when my husband and daughter tested negative, and I realized my only risk was a blood transfusion I had in 1974, 21 years before this test. Even though I had been healthy for two decades, I didn't question what I was told. My intuition told me not to take the AZT that doctors said would cut the chance of me giving HIV to my baby. They finally wore me down, and I started taking AZT in my fifth month.

"After ten months on AZT, I was sick all the time. I had constant diarrhea, nausea, fevers, night sweats and was totally exhausted. I felt like I had a horrible flu that wouldn't go away and I kept developing infections. I was crawling to the bathroom and vomiting for hours. My doctors told me HIV was making me ill, that the virus had mutated into a form that was resistant to AZT, and that I had to go on more drugs to stay alive. Two months after adding 3TC to my treatment regimen, my skin started turning yellow with jaundice. I know that drugs cause jaundice because my father had died of liver failure from heart medicines. Since it was clear that the drugs weren't keeping me from getting AIDS and were actually destroying my liver, I let my prescription run out. I figured I'd rather die from AIDS than liver failure.

"Almost immediately after I stopped taking my medicines—within just a matter of days—I started feeling much better. I had more energy and I wasn't feeling sick. Several months later, all my symptoms disappeared, and I haven't been sick since. I don't think I was ever sick with AIDS, I think I had AZT poisoning. I'm glad that I never gave my daughter Rachel the liquid AZT I was supposed to put in her bottle.

"I took the HIV test twice after Rachel was born and got an indeterminate and a negative result. My daughter is considered a success by medical standards because she tests negative, but I don't care about HIV anymore. I'm concerned about the effects of the AZT she was poisoned with while I was pregnant. Rachel has an enlarged cranium, seizures and a strange deformity near the base of her spine. At age three, still does not speak. I went to this conference on HIV and pregnancy at the Children's Hospital here in Denver. A lot of the mothers there had taken AZT during pregnancy and had their kids with them. Every single one of those kids had enlarged craniums. Their kid's heads looked exactly like Rachel's. They're all AZT babies. I'm working now to repeal Colorado's mandatory testing law."

Kris Chmiel, Denver, CO

"I have been positive, healthy and not on any medicines since being diagnosed positive back in 1984. I can't use my full name as I am a fitness trainer and most people think that HIV=AIDS and leads to death—not exactly good for business!

"I attribute my wellness to refusing doctor's orders, listening to my body and practicing a pretty good diet. Love and support from family help, too."

Jaime P, West Hollywood, CA

"I have been HIV positive since 1983 and decided even then that I wasn't going to let HIV get the better of me. I declined AZT treatment when it was offered early on because I'd watched so many people die while taking it. Instead, I took vitamins, ate properly and worked out.

"In 1987, my partner died and I was overwhelmed with grief. I spent the next five years fighting a serious problem with alcohol addiction. I finally decided that if I didn't get treatment I would die from the alcohol, and I didn't want to go like that.

"In 1996, the AIDS drug cocktails came out and there was such elation, almost hysteria. The new tests were great, the new drugs were great, and everybody was living longer. It was the first good thing to happen in AIDS in the last 15 years. I bought into all the glowing media reports and decided to take the drugs. For a while, I didn't have any side effects except that my cholesterol was rising. After about nine months on the treatments, I started to gain weight, but I looked thinner because my face was getting gaunt. I developed an extended belly, my cheekbones sunk in, and my arms started to waste away. The first time I'd ever felt sick since testing positive was a direct result of taking the medication.

"I got more information about the drugs through HEAL Toronto, and after speaking with Christine Maggiore, one year into the drugs, I decided to quit them. Since then, I've had no problems at all and everything in my body is back to normal. My doctor was annoyed at first, but ultimately he supported my decision. I feel great these days and haven't looked back. I don't go to the gym, but I have a dog and I walk him to the park every day. I tell myself my body is healthy and I'm going to live a long and happy life at least once a day."

Adam Shane, Toronto, Canada

"I was diagnosed HIV positive in the 80s and immediately went into three years of complete denial. I never talked about it or did anything about it. Finally the media campaign HIV=AIDS=Death got to me and I decided it was time to go to an HIV doctor.

"My T cell count was 900; viral load tests were not available then. The doctor put me on AZT, ddI and other medicines. I never questioned the doctor. After approximately two years of taking the HIV drugs, my stomach started getting bloated and I had diarrhea every day. My friend Aaron told me to stop taking the drugs, that they were toxic, but I thought he was crazy.

"Aaron then invited me to attend a meeting in West Hollywood in 1995 where Dr. Peter Duesberg was the speaker. It was too much for me to take in all at once, but one thing stuck in my brain: Dr. Duesberg, a Nobel candidate, affirms that HIV is not the cause of AIDS.

"I took this new information to my HIV doctor. He responded by scaring me with graph after graph showing how HIV was the cause of AIDS. According to his graphs, if I stopped treatment with AZT and the other drugs, I would develop AIDS and die. According to him, those pills were going to enhance the years of life I had left.

"I started to attend the Alive & Well meetings once a month and without telling my doctor, I stopped taking AZT and all the other pills. I then decided it was time to change doctors. I did some research and found an MD that also uses homeopathic treatments. He supported my decision to stop taking the HIV drugs. I then learned about Candida. How come my first doctor never told me anything about it? Within two weeks of doing Candida treatments, my stomach was back to normal and the diarrhea was gone. Now that I was off of the drugs, I started educating myself about nutrition and the immune system. The Alive & Well meetings were very informative and helped me with my research.

"I have been HIV positive and AIDS-free for over 10 years. Now, when I have a health problem, I treat the problem and not HIV. I am very in tune with my immune system. I no longer count my T cells or viral load."

Nick, Beverly Hills, CA

"In May of 1998, I found out that I was pregnant with my first child. I had been seeing the same gynecologist (who is also an obstetrician) for seven years, and she always told me that I had done 'everything right.' I was 29 years old, had been married for six years, took very good care of my health, and had an established career. During a monthly prenatal visit, the nurse said that they would be taking blood. Since I hate needles, I asked why. She told me that they were testing for anemia. A week later I received a frantic phone call from the doctor informing me that I had tested HIV positive. I had no idea that I had even been tested for HIV. I would have never considered myself to be 'at-risk.'

"I was immediately referred to an infectious disease doctor. He tested me again and the result came back positive. He also tested my husband who was inexplicably positive. Although a thorough physical examination failed to show any signs of ill-health—we both felt fine and all our other blood tests, including T cells and viral load, did not indicate otherwise—we were both advised to begin drug therapy. I was told to take AZT for the remainder of my pregnancy while he was told to take the cocktails. Nothing seemed to add up—we have been together for many years, completely monogamous, are exceptionally healthy (my husband runs 4-5 miles a day and competes in marathons) and we have no risk factors. Although the doctors kept promising to 'fill us up with data' my husband and I felt neither comfortable nor convinced.

"These should have been the darkest days of my life, but as serendipity would have it, there was a copy of *What if Everything You Thought You Knew About AIDS Was Wrong?* sitting on our bookshelf that had been sent to us as a gift. I read the book, called members of HEAL, contacted Christine Maggiore, and with their help, began an immediate plan of action that included leaving my doctor of seven years in order to elude the HIV police.

"The result of my otherwise eventless pregnancy is a healthy, happy, breastfed baby girl. I have found a holistic MD who supports our decisions, and our family leads a totally normal life. Normal except for the fear that we could have our daughter taken away from us because of the choices we've made regarding our health. Just last week, the infectious disease specialist who wanted us on the drugs called our home. Once we got the facts, we left his practice and have not seen him for more than a year. He was calling to make sure our family was receiving 'proper treatment.' I'm thankful we were able to avoid falling into a system that would have left us utterly without knowledge of our options.

"I don't know how long my husband and I have been 'HIV positive'—since we met eight years ago? Before that? Since May of 1998? Nothing about our situation makes any sense. The only sense we have found is in the data that shows that most of the ideas we all have about AIDS are wrong."

Stacey Armstrong, Austin, TX

"I'm certain I became HIV positive in December of 1992 because I had the distinct feeling that something happened to me around that time. This feeling was confirmed when I tested HIV positive a few months later. I had just returned to the US from Zimbabwe where I had been living and where I met my husband.

"Since I was already leading a very healthy life, I determined that I would rely on my good health and what I consider our inherent ability to be well rather than following mainstream medical protocol. I don't take drugs. Whether they are pushed on the street or pushed by doctors, drugs are detrimental. I studied what was being said about HIV and AIDS, calculated my risks of becoming ill, and figured I would take my chances and do things my way.

"Initially, I had my T cells monitored regularly. My blood counts have always been on the low side of normal and I'm never sick. I've also been very open about my HIV status and my choices. I think it's important to provide people with another image of what HIV positive means. If I were to accept everything that's said about HIV and AIDS, I would be living as if I were dying. I'm living. Also, as a person of color, it would be suicidal for me to stake my life on a white, male, Western model of medicine. I don't give the medical establishment the power and authority to make decisions for me.

"In 1996, during a trip to Africa, I got malaria. I came home feeling very ill and went to the HIV clinic I frequent for medical care. A doctor there took some blood and without my permission—and with the knowledge I was sick with malaria—ran a T cell count. When the count came back at less than 200, he reported me as an official AIDS case.

"When I found out I was pregnant, I felt certain I could give birth to a healthy baby, but checked in with the clinic doctor for the latest information on drug treatment, AZT and breastfeeding. Although I planned to deliver with a midwife, I asked what would happen if I ended up laboring in a hospital. The answer—12 hours of AZT by IV, a C section, and formula feeding with AZT liquid—sealed my decision to stay out of the system.

"A few months before I was to deliver, I started receiving letters from this doctor that became more threatening as I neared my due date. Even though I replied that I was dealing with my situation in a responsible manner, he reported me to Child Protective Services. When CPS investigators came looking for me, I went to my sister's house. CPS told my mother they wanted to bring her in for questioning, and that they planned to notify the police if she did not cooperate by revealing my whereabouts. Deane Collie of the International Coalition for Medical Justice intervened on my behalf, and was able to convince the CPS not to involve the police or make further threats to my family.

"Ten days after our baby was born at a friend's house, my husband and I packed up our entire lives and fled the state for good. We left behind a home, careers, friends, and family. This is what we have to do to keep our son off toxic AIDS drugs, receiving vital nourishment and immune protection through breastfeeding, and in our custody. As I write this, we have no idea where we are going or what we will do, but at least our son is healthy and in our care."

Katrine Jones, Somewhere in America

"I have been HIV positive and healthy for more than twelve years, without ever having taken AIDS treatments. I first tested positive in 1987.

"I'm a performance artist and writer. A lot of my work challenges conventional ideas about HIV and AIDS. I'm also a former heroin and coke addict. I attribute my good health to stopping those drugs, and ignoring the advice of my doctors to take their drugs instead. If you'd like to know more about my life and my work, email me at fgreen@core.com."

Frank Green, Cleveland, OH

"One of the most devastating experiences of my life was when I found out, in 1992, that my husband had tested HIV positive. The other was when he died in October 1998. He said something that I will carry with me for the rest of my life and it says everything about being diagnosed HIV positive. He said, 'If somebody asked me before this, who are you? I would say I am Cesar, or I am an engineer, or I am Louise's father, or I am Teresa's husband. Now, if somebody asks me, the answer is: I am HIV positive.' Our whole world fell apart. From the minute he was diagnosed, nothing counted anymore. A whole person is defined with three letters, HIV. Everything else vanishes, nothing else is important. Cesar, my husband, died, among other things, of shame.

"One of the first things I decided to do after Cesar tested positive was to call the 800 numbers to get more information on AIDS. I remember the first place I called, I was so desperate that I blurted out: 'I just found out my husband is HIV positive and we have a one-year-old baby. What are our chances of not having it?' The AIDS counselor said: 'Sorry, no chances. You have it and so does your baby.' Can you imagine our despair? Cesar cried, hit his head against the wall and screamed: 'This is the only thing my baby will inherit from me!' At that moment, we decided to kill ourselves, that the only way out would be death. But thinking which one of us would kill Louise, our beautiful baby, stopped us. I later learned that I was not HIV positive then, I am not now, and that our daughter is HIV negative.

"When Cesar and I found out he was positive, we knew only the establishment position. We had never heard about Peter Duesberg, or alternative information, or that there was life after HIV. We were desperate and lived waiting for Cesar's death. After I found Dr. Duesberg and read what he had to say, our lives went back to normal. Our sexual life, and our marriage was like everybody's—we even tried to have another child. My point is not that Duesberg is right—although I am convinced that he is. My point is that the establishment's approach is all wrong. HIV is a matter of faith. It is pure hysteria. The establishment gave us, since the first minute, despair and death.

"Do I think Cesar's immune system was compromised? You bet I do. He was treated with antibiotics since his childhood to prevent diseases, he had many surgeries when he was a little boy, his immune system was destroyed during the course of his life, but not because of HIV. His history was never taken into consideration. Once the doctors found out he was HIV positive, that's what they wanted to treat, nothing else mattered.

"Since Cesar died, our lives—mine and Louise's—changed drastically. We lost many things, among them, our car. When I was cleaning the car, I found a letter in the glove compartment written in hand by Cesar that said if he was not capable to decide for himself, he wanted everybody to know he didn't want to be treated for HIV, he didn't want to take any drugs for the virus. Why did he change his mind? I was right there with him in July of 1998 when the doctor pressured him to take drugs and told him that it would be better for him, that he could live a long life. The doctor never mentioned that Cesar would become paralyzed, that he would have to wear diapers, that he would have unbearable cramps. They waited until he was in the hospital to tell us that his paralysis was the side effect of one of the drugs he was taking. How can a doctor prescribe something whose side effect is paralysis?

"When Cesar took the drugs in 1992, he became very sick and developed many symptoms of AIDS. That's why he stopped taking them—without even knowing there were other opinions about HIV.

"In 1998, the doctor told him that the drugs were different, that they were nothing like they were in 1992 and that he had many patients who were doing well with them. I told Cesar that five years from now that same doctor will be talking to another patient about the new drugs they'll have then. He'll say how bad the drugs were five years before and swear the new ones are completely different.

"I refuse to let Cesar, a whole person, so sensitive, so special, be simply a statistic. He was a whole person, a great human being, that lost everything, including his dignity and his life, because of some people who, in trying to get Nobel prizes and earn fortunes, give the public the wrong information."

Teresa Schmidtz, Miami, FL

"I've been HIV positive for 16 years. I'm a writer and performer, and in my work I emphasize survival and self-determination over the usual death and medical dependency associated with HIV. It's not like I want to second-guess the medical profession, but I have to go with what I know in my heart.

"In the fall of 1996, I came down with PCP pneumonia, one of the hallmark AIDS diseases. I was scared and this was when the cocktails first started coming out, so I decided to try them. I also took drugs for the PCP but when it cleared up, I stopped and just stayed on the cocktail.

"All my numbers were great. My T cells were up, and my viral load was down. But I felt awful. Here I was, a vegetarian who never even took aspirin, and all of a sudden I'm on all these powerful drugs. I had to take pills three or four times a day, some with meals, some without. My whole life revolved around drugs. I was all bloated and kept breaking out into rashes. I had to keep getting up through the night and go to the bathroom, so I was always exhausted. I had horrible neuropathy in my feet to the point where I could hardly walk. I felt my body falling apart, not from HIV, but from the drugs. I was always very aware of my body, and I could feel that I was putting poison into it.

"I finally went to my doctors and told them I didn't want to take the drugs anymore, and they called me a fool. They were very dramatic and told me it was suicide to stop. So instead of stopping, I went on a new combination of drugs. My speech was slurred and I kept losing my equilibrium. When I fell down a flight of stairs at my house, that was the last straw. I just stopped taking them. My T cells went down and my viral load went up, but I felt healthy again. Two years after quitting the treatment, I feel better than ever."

Steven Goldring, Cleveland, OH

"I tested positive in 1989. I've always lived a healthy lifestyle, I don't drink, and I've never done a drug in my life. Due to my antidrug philosophy, I seldom took the medicines offered to me by my doctors, and have never taken any treatments for HIV.

"I have a strong belief, backed up by much documented evidence, that the body, if treated with respect, will take care of itself. But the interesting part of my story is due to the fact that after my initial HIV test which was positive, I subsequently tested negative, then once again positive, and then negative.

"I will not take another HIV test due to its highly inaccurate and unreliable results, which even the *New England Journal of Medicine* notes as being nonspecific and open to interpretation. I have never suffered from anything other than common flu and colds, and even once bacterial pneumonia. I've always been healthy with the exception of the illnesses I have mentioned. To anyone who's tested positive I would like to say: Take control of your life. Educate yourself to the facts like I did and become another long-term survivor!"

Greg Drolette, Los Angeles, CA

"I tested HIV positive on August 20, 1985. My doctor's clientele were mostly children and babies, so she had some fears about continuing to see me in her office. She was concerned particularly about airborne HIV so she shuffled me off to another doctor. A nice message to my subconscious that I am a dangerous person.

"His treatment was a combination of vitamin C injections and heparin as he thought this would prevent a further decline of the T cell helper-suppressor ratio. I went along with this for a few months. However, I had never looked favorably on drugs and decided to stop the treatment. All the while, I was being fed the negativity of how fatal this virus was by my lover and my doctor. I was having lots of canker sores in my mouth along with chronic fatigue. Then one day something clicked and I realized I needed to get away from this negative input. So I dropped my doctor and my lover, and was soon doing quite well. This really brought home to me how much fear and negativity impact one's health.

"Around mid-1995, I left the AIDS clinic where I had been going. Although I was continually being pressured by the nurses and physicians to start some kind of drug therapy, this was not the reason I left. I left because I was twice refused treatment because my condition was not HIV-related. I found this quite annoying as I've always been of the opinion that you treat the whole person and don't refuse needed treatment because it falls outside of some category.

"Soon after this, I was thrilled to discover that I was not alone in the struggle to deal with this HIV phenomenon. In early 1997, I found a doctor who was open to alternative treatment and agreed not to push drug treatment on me or push the prevailing HIV hypothesis. She does not necessarily agree with my views but she's very clear that you must respect your patient's views. She also teaches at a medical school and periodically invites me to speak to new medical students about my views on HIV and AIDS. She wants them to develop the same attitude and to help them see that prevailing medical doctrine is to be questioned.

"I am doing just fine after over 14 years. It took me some time to realize that I'm not going to die prematurely. One of the hardest things of this whole HIV mess is seeing so many friends die. In 1995 I lost nine, supposedly from AIDS. All of them insisted on doing the various drug therapies despite my efforts to dissuade them. One person who I tried to talk to says he very much believes in Western medicine and that one's belief is the senior thing; that's why drugs work for him and not taking drugs works for me. I say, if it's a matter of belief, who would choose a belief where you have to take toxic drugs?"

Andy Swenson, Silverlake, CA

"I was a long term heroin addict for some 20 years. I started using as a teenager and come from the school of 'just say yes!' to any and all drugs. Well, one day in 1985 I'm at work as a carpenter and I fall off a roof and break my back, pelvis, wrist, and other bones. I was in a lot of pain so the doctor wanted to administer Demerol when I told him that I'm an addict who has a resistance to opiates. As a result, I got—without my knowledge—an HIV test. Two or three days later, while in traction, I'm suddenly moved out of my hospital room and put in an isolation room. I'm alone now and everyone begins to wear masks and rubber gloves when they enter. Is there any need to mention how that made me feel? My employer receives a document from his insurance company that tells him I'm HIV positive. So much for confidentiality regarding my health status. I'm so ashamed that I never return to work, besides my boss doesn't want me around because of my 'condition.' No better excuse does a person without the highest self-esteem need to continue down the self-destructive path of addiction, especially because now I was definitely going to die. The man in the white lab coat told me so...

"Fast-forward to November 1992. I'm in a drug and alcohol rehab center and a volunteer gives me a photocopy of Celia Farber's 1991 article in *SPIN* magazine 'Fatal Distraction.' That was the beginning of the rest of my life. I began spitting out my AZT. I began a journey of recovery from addiction.

"The medical clinic I went to early in my sobriety told me I was just 'lucky' to be as healthy as I was because I refused to take their damn drugs. I have a holistic physician who has given me some IV vitamin therapy to restore some vital nutrients to my system—20 years of alcohol and drug abuse will deplete your immunity and your nutrient levels. I've been married four years now, am completely healthy at age 49, and in better shape than ever before in my life. I've been a vegetarian for six years and volunteer in rehab but they won't allow me to share the truth about HIV in that forum...something about it being against the law, so I do the best I can anywhere I can with the information.

"I have taken responsibility for my own life and have not allowed someone in a white lab coat do it for me. Had I chosen that path they offered me, I know I would be dead. I'm a survivor because someone had the guts to tell me the truth about the HIV=AIDS=Death lie. It's bad science in the hands of bad government."

Scott Zanetti, Morristown, NJ

"After using heroin for four years, I went for an extended stay in Mexico to deal with my addiction. After successfully giving up heroin, I came home. Later, in 1987, I tested HIV positive. At the time, my T cell count was 400 and my doctor was very pessimistic about the future. Instead of giving up, I decided to make a longtime dream of going hiking in the Himalayas come true. It was 1988.

"When I returned from Nepal, my T cell count was 1220 and my doctor was completely baffled. I began to explore homeopathy. After a period of good health, in 1990, I began to feel very tired. My doctor insisted, in spite of my high T cell count, that it was because of HIV. I changed my diet to organic foods even though throughout all of this, I was repeatedly pressured to go on AZT. Finally, I was diagnosed with hepatitis B. I stopped drinking alcohol and, in 1991, went to India and began a curative diet of fruits and coconut milk. After regaining my strength and returning home at the end of summer, I discovered that I was pregnant. Again, I was pressured to take AZT. I was also pressured to abort. I refused. My baby was born HIV positive and following the birth, my T cell count was very low and I was exhausted. Although I was continually pressured to expose my baby to numerous tests and to give him AZT, I declined. One year later, I consented to having my baby tested a second time. He tested HIV negative.

"Although I have had other health challenges since, I treat each problem individually and live a full life in France with my son and husband. It has been 13 years since I tested HIV positive."

Sylvie Cousseau, Paris, France

"In October 1990, we adopted a little girl born in Romania when she was just a few days old. When we brought her to America two months later, Lilly was a happy, healthy baby. We took her for a complete medical exam that included an HIV test. The result was positive, and although she had no symptom of illness, she was immediately put on AZT syrup and Septra, a powerful antibiotic. We investigated and discovered that her birth mother tested HIV negative. This information seemed not to matter, we were told Lilly had the 'AIDS virus.' For close to a year, we gave her AZT and other drugs, until by the grace of God, we determined that the drugs were making her very ill.

"During her first 18 months on the drugs, Lilly's health declined. She was hyperactive, almost as though she didn't feel comfortable in her body. She didn't eat properly and suffered nausea and diarrhea and fell behind in growth rate. Doctors attributed her problems to HIV and increased the dosage. A few months later, her doctor began pressuring us to add ddI to our daughter's drug regimen. She praised Lilly's progress at each visit even though by then Lilly had completely stopped growing and her T cells were dropping. Then for three months in 1992, Lilly woke up in the middle of the night grabbing her knees and screaming in pain. We took her to the University of Minnesota after the screaming bouts started. The doctor barely acknowledged what we were saying and left us with the impression 'Well what do you expect? This kid is dying of AIDS.'

"In desperation, we turned to Dr. Peter Duesberg, a source we had previously discounted. We had read a couple articles about Duesberg but never gave his views serious consideration; now we wrote to him at UC Berkeley asking for advice. He responded promptly with a package of literature and we started researching for ourselves.

"Almost immediately we understood our daughter's problem was not an immune deficiency, but the side-effects of drugs. We took her off them and have not looked back since. Two days after we stopped the AZT, her leg cramps stopped. She started sleeping much better and began eating two to three times as much as she had ever eaten before. We found a doctor who uses a holistic approach to disease that puts a big emphasis on nutrition. After two months of nutritional therapy, she started gaining weight. By 27 months of age, she was back in the 10th percentile of growth.

"When we tried to discuss our decision to stop AZT with the MD at the university and put Lilly's real progress in perspective, we were verbally attacked and treated as if we were children. We didn't tell the doctor that Lilly was off the drugs that day. Instead, we sent a letter. Her response was to threaten to have Lilly removed from our home. She said that taking her off AZT would hasten her decline and death, and that there are foster homes for children whose parents don't go along with the medical community.

"Eight years later, Lilly is a perfectly healthy little girl. She does well in school, has lots of friends, enjoys riding her bike and is an avid swimmer."

Scott and Cathy Norton, Minneapolis, Minnesota

"If you had told me five years ago that I would believe that HIV didn't cause AIDS, that I'd question AIDS drugs, I'd have thought you were crazy. I had a lover for seven years who was diagnosed positive and he took the treatment at the time which was AZT monotherapy. Knowing what we know now about AZT, I really believe that's what killed him. And as he sat on his deathbed, I think that's what he was thinking, too, because he begged me to take him off the drugs. But because I believed that dying from HIV would be more horrendous than from any toxic side effect, I encouraged him to stay on the drugs. I now want to stop this insidious death ritual where people, out of caring and compassion, are administering death to their loved ones.

"If you take out a liter of my blood, you can't find any virus, you can only find antibodies. I learned in Biology 101 that the body produces antibodies to kill things like a virus. If you can't find the virus and you can find antibodies, why can I not conclude that my body has done the job it's designed to do? That if I test positive on an HIV test, it is not a result of immune suppression, but in fact a sign of a normal immune reaction?

"Everyone who tests positive should be told that not taking AIDS treatments is a healthy option. I've had an AIDS diagnosis for 5 years based on having 180 T cells and a viral load of 350,000. According to their rules, I should be on my deathbed. I'm not even close.

"We are consistently being told that it is unethical for drug researchers to conduct studies using placebo groups—people who test HIV positive and are not on the drugs. But when studies just compare drugs to drugs, AZT to AZT and protease inhibitors, then there's no recognition of people who aren't on any drugs. What are they studying?

"The HIV hypothesis is not a theoretical debate. As a member of ACT UP, I speak out about this because I'm trying to save lives. I feel I perpetuated AIDS. I stood in front of Harvard Medical Center and demanded the release of ddI and ddC. I wonder how many people I harmed with my AIDS activism. And I'm really trying to figure out what my life has been devoted to. I feel we need to get to the bottom of this and put an end to the madness."

Michael Bellefountaine, San Francisco, CA

"When I tested HIV positive 16 years ago, the road map for how to die with this condition seemed clear. Creating my own path has been challenging and rewarding. HIV has been a catalyst for personal growth, an inspiration to make changes I needed to make anyway. My life is richer as a result.

"Although I deal with fear all the time, I never really internalized the HIV=AIDS=Death dogma. I instinctively believed that HIV was a cofactor and that I could manage my health successfully without drug therapies. I pursue an aggressive health management program that includes nutrition and supplementation, exercise and appropriate rest. I use Western, naturopathic and traditional Chinese medicine on an as-needed basis.

"While I tend to my body with attention and dedication, I know that all healing is ultimately healing of the spirit. For this reason, I am devoted to my spiritual practice. I choose to put my faith in the power of God to heal me rather than in the power of a virus to destroy me."

Duncan MacLachlan, Toronto, Canada

"In March of 1997, I woke up with a rash on my hands and feet that became so painful and intense, it was totally unbearable. I went to see the doctor I've had since I left my pediatrician. He said I was having an allergic reaction and that it would pass. As long as I was in his office, and since I had just broken up with my girlfriend of three years, I asked him to do an HIV test. I figured that there was no way I was positive—I had tested negative three years ago when I went into the relationship that just ended, and I didn't have any experiences that put me 'at risk.'

"I got a call from the nurse a few days later inviting me to come in and talk to the doctor. She tried to sound casual but her tone made my heart drop. It was obvious something was very wrong. I had to demand to speak to the doctor before she would put me through to him. He told me not to worry, that there had been 'a glitch' in my HIV test and we had to do it again. Once I was in his office, he explained the 'glitch.' He said it was like my car had a full tank of gas but there was a glitch in the gas gauge that made the needle point to empty even though my car was full for sure because I'd just filled it. After this highly technical explanation, he took my blood for another test. As I left he told me 'I'm 99% positive that you're negative. The tests are unreliable.' I took him at his word.

"Three days later, the nurse called again with the same invitation to see the doctor, but this time, no matter what I said, she wouldn't put the doctor on the phone. When I saw my doctor, he told me that the HIV test looks for eight proteins that the body produces when a person become infected, and that if the test finds five or more, a person is HIV positive. He said that my first test had one positive and four negative proteins; the second one had two positive, one indeterminate, and two negative proteins. When I asked what the proteins were, he said they were antibodies, and he used chicken pox antibodies as an example. I asked him why antibodies meant I was immune from chicken pox but that I had HIV. He said HIV was different and I believed him. I had a lot of faith in my doctor. He took my blood again and told me to come back in three days with one of my parents.

"My doctor later told us that breaking the news about my positive test was the hardest thing he had to do in the last ten years of his practice. I cried, my dad cried, the doctor cried. I was 21 years old and it was all over. In a few seconds, my life expectancy went from 85 years to 25.

"While I thought about how to live out my final years, my dad concentrated on getting me the best care money had to offer. He flew Martin Delaney, the head of the AIDS treatment group Project Inform, in from San Francisco to meet with me in our living room. Marty said it was imperative I start the drugs immediately. After that, I was brought to doctors at UCLA. Since my risks couldn't be identified, they supposed I was gay and simply unwilling to admit it, and went looking for evidence by sticking glove-covered fingers in my rectum. They, too, said I needed to 'hit it early and hard' with the drugs. Next, my dad and I were on a plane to New York to meet with Dr. David Ho, the AIDS researcher who had recently been named *Time* magazine's Man of the Year. After that, I took a week off from AIDS research. The only decision left to make was which drug regimen to begin, when my ex-girlfriend called.

"I was not at all into hearing anymore about HIV and AIDS from her or other friends with good intentions, but I had a feeling I needed to listen. One thing I've learned from this experience is to honor my intuition. She told me that I had to see her friend Laura the next day, and somehow I knew that when Laura walked through the door with two shopping bags full of books, my life was about to change. After one book, I realized that my doctor had no idea what was going on and that with just this information, I already knew more than him. A few more books later, I was questioning what Delaney and Ho had to say.

"Then I went to see Christine Maggiore. She was so calm, it kind of bugged me. After I read her book, it was all over. I read some more just to solidify my knowledge, and so I would be ready with the facts when faced with the inevitable, 'But don't you see you're in denial?' Knowing what I know now, there is no way I would ever take the drugs. I have just one more year before I beat the prognosis of the UCLA doctors who told me, based on my T cells and viral load, to expect illness in three to five years. Instead of being ill, I surf every day that there are waves, I do yoga, I eat organic foods and meditate. I love being alive; life is truly beautiful.

"My father has gone from hysterical and heartbroken about my decisions, to learning to trust me a little more. My whole family is still afraid for me, but a least they're listening. People can't really say much when you have the facts. Not even Martin Delaney and David Ho."

Randy Harman, Malibu, CA

"When I first heard of Gay Related Immune Deficiency (GRID) in 1983, the media reports were already talking about an infectious disease. I thought how ridiculous—viruses aren't brainy enough to pick out the gays from the straights! Simplistic as that reaction may seem to me now, I think it was fundamentally a valid intuition. My time for an 'HIV test' came in 1985 when an amorous encounter called me and I landed in a doctor's office for a Hepatitis B test. Antibodies? Yes. A further test for infection showed no infection, but the doctor wasn't done with me yet.

"I'll never forget how things played out at the tropical disease clinic where my HIV antibody tests were run. My first result was negative. I remember stumbling over the semantic flip-flop for a moment: Negative is good, isn't it? Because I had a few slightly inflamed lymph nodes and my 'risk status,' the doctors doubted the negative result. More blood was drawn.

Two weeks later, I was given a positive result. No doubts among the doctors this time. I said 'OK, how about two outta three? And you must have some other test, like with Hepatitis B, to see if my antibodies have done the job and cleared the infection...' I was told that the clinic was backed up with requests for HIV tests and that I might call my doctor for retesting in six months, but for now I should consider myself infected.

"That confusing and contradictory experience left me highly skeptical. In the past 15 years, I've made some unconventional choices—I've never touched any 'anti-HIV' drugs or alternative 'AIDS therapies.' I subscribe to an 'If it ain't broke, don't fix it' philosophy and I avoid doctors. I'm also convinced that Queers will never live free as long as we are afraid to deconstruct the epidemic of hysteria called AIDS."

Robert Johnston, Toronto, Canada

"I remember the day I received my positive result like it was yesterday. I figured I'd test positive since I'd had unprotected sex with a couple of guys I later learned had died from AIDS. I really thought that I was prepared to hear the result. Nothing could have been further from the truth. I sobbed uncontrollably all the way home. I felt like I had become a character in some sci-fi movie with an alien thing growing inside me that would come bursting out of my chest as I died a horrific death. A part of me did die that day, the part that dreamed and looked towards the future.

"Denial lasted for over a year. I wasn't ready to start thinking about dying so I just ignored the whole thing. It wasn't until I started dating someone else who was positive that I started thinking about trying to fight this thing inside me.

"My new love was a nurse who worked for a doctor who specialized in AIDS treatment. When I began a new job that provided medical benefits I started seeing this doctor and after a confirmatory antibody test I was put on regimen AZT and Zovirax. I tried to be a good little pill popper for a while but I grew weary of the little beeping pill box and soon I was missing my meds half the time. The doctors reduced the dosage about a year later and then I became even more irregular with my meds. About two years later, I tested positive a third time and AZT and Zovirax were prescribed again even though my T cells were still a healthy 600 plus.

"Given that I knew I wasn't taking my meds regularly I began to wonder if I was really sick since my T cells remained so stable with or without the drugs. For the next three years I took all my pills in the morning if I remembered and would go six months or more without them if I ran out. I'd worry that my next blood test would show that my T cells were dropping but this was never the case. I know now that a part of my lack of discipline came from the fact that I had already given up on the rest of my life. Looking forward was just too painful. Planning for the future seemed pointless. I never really made a conscious decision to stop taking the meds. I just never went back to get more pills the last time they ran out.

"A little over a year ago, an acquaintance introduced me to *Inventing the AIDS Virus* by Peter Duesberg. I went out and bought the book and read it cover to cover in a single sitting. As the sun rose that morning, I sobbed for hours. Then I became angry. Since then I have been reading everything I can get my hands on about the controversy surrounding the HIV=AIDS=Death hypothesis.

"Today, I am actually able to look towards my future with hope. The nagging fear is hard to shake off, especially when you're married to a healthcare worker who still finds it hard to believe all those doctors and scientists could be wrong. Everyday I seem farther from the fear and more excited about the possibilities of growing old—12 years ago I didn't think I would make it to 40."

Michael Davis, Topanga, CA

"I was in a monogamous relationship from 1981 to 1992. After the relationship ended in 92, I tested HIV positive. My former partner is HIV negative. He and I remain good friends because our relationship is built on trust. The HIV counselor insisted our relationship must not have been monogamous. Looking back, I think that because my situation did not follow the model for HIV, they were trying to change my circumstances to fit their rules. Since my former partner tests negative, how could HIV be a sexually transmitted disease?

"Testing positive for HIV antibodies changed my life. I was scared that I would get AIDS and die within two years. Once the news of my HIV status became common knowledge among my friends, I noticed a drastic change in their behavior towards me. They became overly sympathetic, like there was something wrong with me. Most of my friends who took the test for HIV antibodies came up negative. Knowing this only compounded my despair and hopelessness. They would make comments like 'Ron, you look so well.'

"My first T cell count was 500 which, in 1992, put me on the border line for AZT treatment. The Northwest AIDS Foundation showed me a graph demonstrating how I could expect my T cell counts to drop and continue to go down. Because I had a strong will to live, I decided to eliminate stress in my life by stepping down from a middle management position to a staff position. I avoided people who offered me little hope or encouragement while I was dealing with my health crisis. To counter the negativity around me, I would think positive thoughts like living a long, productive life. I would envision myself climbing hills and mountains, and my T cell counts gradually increasing. As a result, I had sequential T cell counts in the 900s.

"In June of 1994, I ran across an interview with Jon Rappoport, the author of *AIDS Inc.*, in the *Seattle Common Ground*. Finding information that challenged my ideas about AIDS set me on a path of discovery which led me to people who not only helped me, but who made it possible for me to help others.

"I learned that the HIV tests detect antibodies formed in response to the virus, not the virus itself, and that the antibodies detected may not even be due to infection with HIV. Because of cross-reactions with antibodies produced by the hepatitis B vaccination, which I had been given, and many other microbes, there was no way to know what my positive test result meant.

"Almost eight years after testing positive, I remain in good health. I do not monitor my T cell count and viral load, and don't follow mainstream medical protocol. Instead, I see a naturopathic doctor and acupuncturist. I live in a loving household with my new boyfriend and two dogs. I reach out to others through *HEAL Naturally*, a public access TV show I produce which operates as a project under the Gay Community Social Services."

Ron Piazza, Seattle, Washington

"In 1989, when I was 21 years old, I went to the local health department for a pregnancy test. They asked me if they should include an HIV test, and I agreed. About two weeks later, I got a call at work from a health department employee who told me my pregnancy test was negative, but my HIV test was indeterminate, and that I had to test again. A few days after I took a second test, the health department called and said I had to come back in, but this time I couldn't get any information over the phone. Once I was there, I was told that I had tested HIV positive.

"All I remember of that two hour appointment is this counselor drawing circles on a paper. He drew a circle to represent an immune cell and explained that HIV made the circle explode, unleashing all these other little circles of HIV that would infect other immune cells and make those explode. I left the health department in hysterics and called my parents. I went home and told my boyfriend that I had tested positive. He accused me of giving him AIDS.

"I figured I had two years to live at the most. I based this on the famous AIDS victim Kimberly Bergalis, a healthy young woman who lived just two years after testing HIV positive, and my own history of poor health. When I was 13 years old, I was diagnosed with rheumatoid arthritis. When I was 18, I started having stomach problems. After many doctor visits and medications, I had surgery to remove my appendix and a few inches of my colon. After that, I was diagnosed with Crohn's disease, an incurable intestinal disorder. I was told this disease would compromise my immune system and give me constant stomach pain for the rest of my life. During the next two years, I came down with mononucleosis, chicken pox, stomach ulcers, and chronic fatigue.

"By the time I tested positive, I was already frustrated with the medical treatments I had been on for Crohn's disease and the doctors were pushing me to take steroids, which I was unwilling to do. Instead, I found a book on Crohn's from a health food store and started on an alternative plan. I began taking acidophilus for my stomach and went through a detoxification using blue-green algae. At the same time as the detox, I began to focus on strengthening my immune system, knowing intuitively that this was the way to go. For five years, I made slow but certain progress with my health using a wide range of herbs, vitamins and minerals. For the past three years, despite my dismal medical history and my positive HIV diagnosis, I have wonderful, vibrant energy which makes me feel so fortunate. I have had no stomach pain for about five years. Interestingly, my T cell counts have never varied—in sickness and in health, they are always about 700.

"In 1998, I had an unexpected blessing—I discovered I was pregnant with twins. I found an excellent doctor at a well-known hospital who I thought would help me find the best way to ensure the health of my children. Instead, he said he was unable to advise me about HIV, and sent me to what he described as one of the best HIV specialists in the country. This turned out to be a run-down, dirty hospital where social workers kept me waiting in lines for hours. A social worker gave me coverage for medication costs and told me that I should start medication right away, before I had even seen a doctor or had a viral load test. I walked out completely frustrated.

"In the fifth month of my pregnancy, my whole life changed. I learned of Christine Maggiore and the work that she was doing. She told me everything I needed to hear and followed up with articles, studies, books, videos, and other information—I lost count of all the packages she sent—which I carefully read and studied. It became clear that the only way to avoid AZT and a Cesarean section was to have a midwife-assisted home birth. Ironically, after thorough research on home births, I became convinced this was the safest and most pleasing environment to birth my children.

"I had two midwives and two assistants for my home birth. There were no complications or medical interventions. At no point did I question that I had made the right choice. I carried the girls to the 40th week with a high protein nutritional program, and was active until the birth. This is unexpected in a multiple pregnancy handled by medical doctors who often recommend bed rest in the last several weeks. Together the twins weighed in at over 12 pounds. They are healthy, beautiful and gaining weight appropriately. An awesome accomplishment for a pregnancy with so much additional stress. I often wonder where we would be today if I hadn't discovered the many alternatives to the HIV=AIDS=Death views. Don't let a doctor or health officials tell you what you have to do without knowing your options. Life is so precious!"

Lynn C, Lake Tahoe, Nevada

"On May 31, 1991 I had my second daughter who is now eight years old. Following the delivery, the hospital gave me what they described as a standard blood test for women who have just given birth. A week later, I got a call from my doctor who told me that I was HIV positive. At the same time, she stated that my test 'was unclear.' She offered no other information except a referral to a specialist. The doctor she referred me to tested me again and said this new test came out positive, but that he was 80% sure I was a 'false positive.' He then did a Western Blot which he claimed was more sensitive. When that test came back, he could not give me a straight answer; he only said, 'Let's assume at this point you have it.'

"You cannot imagine the mental torture that I went through being told congratulations, you are the proud mother of a beautiful little girl, but you will not be able to watch her grow up. I was 21 years old and suddenly my life was over. The torture continued as they explained that my baby might have contracted HIV from me. For two years, they gave my daughter HIV tests; some were positive and some were negative. At the age of two, she had three tests in a row come back with a negative result. Wanting never to put another child through this, I had surgery to ensure I could never again become pregnant.

"Even though I had no detectable viral load and had no symptoms of AIDS, in 1997 they put me on a combination of 36 pills a day. Within a couple days of starting the cocktail, I began to lose strength and feel tired all the time. I developed stomach problems, pain mostly, and lost my appetite. The doctor told me that starting the medication early, before symptoms developed, would increase my life span. Before I started the medication my T cell count was over 1,200 and I had an undetectable viral load. Two months into the medication, besides feeling sick all the time, my T cell had count dropped to below 500. My instinct told me that this was not OK so I stopped the cocktail. I am thankful I only took the medications for a couple of months. My doctor told me many times that I am a long-term survivor while at the same time, he and other doctors kept trying to get me to try other medications.

"In July of 1997, I met my current husband, David Anderson. I told him about having tested HIV positive when we first stated dating. Dave refused to believe that nothing could be done and began to research HIV and AIDS. One day while searching the internet, Dave found Professor Peter Duesberg's website. Through this site he found others such as Alive & Well and HEAL, and he began to make contact with people from both sides of the argument that HIV causes AIDS. We carefully read all materials published by pharmaceutical companies who manufacture anti-HIV drugs. For a year and a half, we read medical journals, research papers, and interviews. Dave and I concluded that AIDS is caused by something other than HIV. Our conclusion is based on the lack of evidence for HIV and the lack of answers to basic questions. The only hard evidence we came up with is that drugs cause AIDS, and that a positive HIV test could be the result of many things such as flu, pregnancy, cancer, and other things I have experienced. Moreover, HIV testing is not standardized, that is, you can test positive at one lab and negative at another. It would be nice if all diseases could be cured just by changing labs.

"I do not see a doctor regarding my diagnosis nor do I consume any antiviral medications. Eight and a half years after testing positive, I am healthier than ever. I am 29, have a wonderful husband and have two healthy girls. This is not to say all is well simply because I have found a new reality. My oldest daughter, who is 11 years old, lives with my parents. Her father died in 1989 in an earthquake and my parents took temporary guardianship over her. My HIV positive diagnosis has been used in preventing me from getting her back in my custody. Also, ever since testing positive, I've been struggling with anxiety attacks. Despite these attacks, I am going to live my life happy and drug-free."

Rhonda Anderson, Austin, TX

"I was diagnosed HIV positive in 1990. In 1994, protease inhibitors had yet to be licensed for use. Although I had no symptoms of illness, I was encouraged to join a clinical trial which was the only way to access them. At the end of this two-year trial, the drugs would be made available to everyone if they worked, but the way they were being heralded as a 'marvelous new treatment,' or even a possible cure for AIDS, it was as if it was a forgone conclusion that they worked. It was like I was being granted an enormous favor by this early access.

"If I'd known the facts, I would have never agreed to be in the trial, but I didn't. And after all, I thought, doctors know best. So in March of 1995, I agreed to take part. The trial consisted of AZT, ddI and Saquinavir, a protease inhibitor. Neither I nor the hospital knew if I was on the drugs or the placebo (which was actually AZT monotherapy) and my viral load results were only revealed to the pharmaceutical company. Immediately upon starting the trial, my T cell count plummeted and remained at the same low level. At the end of the two years, it was revealed that I'd been on AZT monotherapy for the first six months, and then on all three drugs for the remainder of the trial. If someone had asked me then if I'd suffered any side effects, the answer would have been no but now I know otherwise. During the first year, I needed a blood transfusion. During the second year I developed lipodystrophy—I had a paunch, my upper arms became thinner, and the veins of my lower limbs began to protrude. But at the time, I put this down to my imagination.

"By 1997, the clinic possessed an entire menu of drugs and therefore decided to change my combination to Ritonovir, 3TC and D4T and they could do their own viral load testing. My count was 24,000, relatively low, so the doctor assumed that my load must have been incredibly high at the beginning of the trial. Instead, when the trial results were released, they showed I had fluctuated at a constantly low level.

"I had concerns about the new drugs, especially Ritonovir, after having read in *Rolling Stone* magazine that some people had died of liver failure while taking it. My doctor brushed aside these concerns as if I were crazy for even raising them. He did, however, warn me to expect dire side effects for the first two weeks. Ironically, the side effects began after two weeks—numbing and tingling in the lips, burning sensation in my upper arms, lethargy, insomnia, crippling stomach cramps and chronic diarrhea. Admittedly, these would mostly occur within a few hours of taking the drugs. The rest of the time, I would be reasonably fine. Then the diarrhea became uncontrollable. The doctor blamed a parasite, but my tests came back clear. He assured me the diarrhea would stop after six weeks. It did not.

"'It is important to restore a person's quality of life' says one of the ads for the drugs. Well, all they succeeded in doing to me was to decimate any quality that I had possessed. I no longer had the energy to go to the gym or to participate in regular social activities. I wasn't even able to go out due to toilet problems—I lost count of the designer underwear I ruined. The practicalities of taking the drugs at certain times, with meals, with liquids, also made conducting a normal life impossible. I spent my days watching cable TV and popping pills which only added to my feelings of depression and isolation.

"As my viral load stubbornly refused to go down to undetectable, the doctor decided to reintroduce Saquinavir. Combining it with Ritonovir was said to increase its absorption 40 times, and even though no one knew what effect this would have, they added it to my treatment regimen. I developed a skin abscess that swelled to the size of a golf ball and then burst.

"The pills now filled me with dread. I had a strong intuitive feeling they were killing me which conflicted with the rhetoric of my doctor and the pharmaceutical companies. I felt confused and frightened with no one to turn to. I felt like I was constantly being fed only one side of the story.

"Despite all the efforts to portray the drugs as marvelous and wonderful, other information came seeping through—accounts of the mounting side effects and of people dying while on the drugs, along with the true reasons why people with AIDS were living long and what the real causes of AIDS were. I realized that I had been denied the basic right to an informed decision. I began a relentless quest for the truth. When I found out that the viral load test—the only thing that gives any credence to the drugs—basically picks up scraps of genetic material and amplifies the result, I lost all faith in the drugs and my fear was replaced with anger. I made the decision to stop taking the drugs.

"Within weeks I felt better. The diarrhea stopped, the skin abscesses went away, the stomach cramps disappeared, and my T cells shot up. I realized that I had become so used to the effects of the drugs that my ill health had become an accepted state of being, and that I was unaware of the damage being done. I think many people taking the drugs who say they are doing well may be as unaware as I was of the destruction taking place within their own body.

"At the final visit with my doctor, I lacked the courage to tell him I'd stopped the drugs, afraid he might berate me. Then fate intervened—my last viral load, taken prior to stopping the drugs, had shot up dramatically. He took this as a sign that the drugs were no longer working and failed to take into consideration the fact that I'd had the flu when the test was performed. Despite the facts I now knew, I kept quiet. I breathed a sigh of relief knowing the doctor would make the decision to take me off the drugs. The relief soon turned to despair when he announced he wanted to put me on a combination of five different drugs. I never saw the doctor again.

"It cannot be said that the drugs were responsible for 'keeping me well' for the three years I took them, as the doctor would like me to believe. My first two years on the drugs had been in a trial utilizing a combination that has since been deemed ineffective, and during the final year, I had been plagued with ill health. If anything, I am now well in spite of the drugs, not because of them.

"The decision to stop taking the drugs is a difficult one in the face of pressure from doctors, the propaganda from the pharmaceutical companies and the organizations funded by them, and all the media hype. You really have to believe in yourself and take responsibility for your own life out of their hands and into your own, and just let go. Like Dumbo the elephant who believed he couldn't fly without the aid of a feather, once he let go, he realized that he could fly without it. Once you take that leap of faith you realize there is life without the drugs."

Stephen Rogers, London, England

"In 1970, 11 years before the emergence of AIDS and 14 years before Gallo's discovery of HIV, I began to experience the first signs of immune collapse. It started with a persistent flu that lasted seven months and left me so nauseous and aching I could hardly function. A series of doctors told me that my symptoms were impossible, that a flu lasts weeks, not months, and they advised I go home and rest. Eventually I recovered. But then the impossible happened again.

"I wasn't able to mount a challenge to most any ordinary bug. It was very frightening because I realized that I was sinking lower and lower. I would go to doctors and tell them that something must be wrong with my immune system. But since this was years before the immune system became the focus of medical research, they treated me like I was nuts for even bringing up the idea. Because no tests they gave me ever revealed what was wrong, they would act annoyed when I would present myself again. 'We told you there's nothing wrong with you and now you're back.' When I tried to make this point about the immune system, they would roll their eyes and act as if I had said something totally bizarre.

"I began to live in terror of winter and the flu. For years, I restricted my activities and avoided crowds. Despite my extreme efforts, in 1988 I became ill again and this time I didn't recover. I collapsed at work—I don't even recall how I got home—and went to bed for the next five years. In rapid succession I developed several of what I later learned were the cardinal signs of AIDS: oral thrush, wasting syndrome (which took me down to 78 pounds), diarrhea, fatigue, and dementia to the degree that I sometimes could not make out if people were actually speaking to me and if they were, what they were saying; words in books would appear as meaningless marks.

"On one of my good days, I made it to the bathroom by myself, and curious about a strange sensation in my mouth and throat, I looked in the mirror. My tongue was covered with a thick white growth, thick enough to cut with scissors. This sight inspired me to call a nutritionist someone had recommended—after being dismissed and even laughed at by doctors, I had given up asking them for help. In three minutes on the phone with her I learned that I had systemic candidiasis, a sign of a very depleted immune system, and that the constant illnesses I had were opportunistic infections typical of AIDS. What was left for me to discover was how I could have all these AIDS-defining illnesses even though I am in no AIDS risk group. According to the HIV/AIDS construct, there was no explanation for my depleted immune system.

"The nutritionist put me on a program of natural antifungal remedies, but my case was too far gone to respond. In 1992, I was passed on to an MD who miraculously knew what he was doing. He treated me in such a way that my immune system was able to regenerate itself. But it took a long time and I nearly died before I got better. About 12 months after I started the antifungal program, I actually got out of the house for the first time in years—a very shaky little walk to the corner grocery store. It's still hard for me to remember what great health is like, but mine is improving continually.

"I discovered that there is a lot of semantic confusion about AIDS. If you take immune suppression at face value, then it becomes much more logical, and the risks cover a broader area than the official CDC categories. The major risk for me was constant exposure to toxic chemicals through my skin and lungs in the course of my work as an artist—paint thinners, vaporizing chemicals, acids and inks that I've since found out are some of the most toxic substances with which one can work. For years, I was practically bathing in these chemicals. Several courses of antibiotics, along with taking birth control pills, and cortisone injections for recurring yeast infections just worsened my condition.

"I don't think it is unreasonable to say that if you start out life with an intact immune system and find yourself midway through with one that has been destroyed, this qualifies as AIDS—no matter how it was destroyed. The body cannot know whether it is being dosed with toxins in the course of one's work, taking them in as pharmaceuticals while under the care of a doctor, or while dancing the night away under the influence of designer drugs. There are many roads that lead to toxic overload—even the emotional toxicity of being told you carry a fatal virus.

"I support Peter Duesberg 100% in his toxicity/AIDS hypothesis because of my own experience. I feel as though I have been, very unwillingly, conducting a scientific experiment in my own body. I didn't have to find any strange virus to explain my illness and I didn't have to wait for the development of drugs to recover. My immune collapse didn't happen because I had sex with the wrong person, it happened because a body exposed to an onslaught of toxic substances, for whatever reason, will eventually break down. Unfortunately, the medical industry does not want to divorce itself from the germ theory, from the 'single-cause theory,' and look at the wider picture. If studies were funded to investigate the effects of toxins on the immune system, I think that the 'mystery' of AIDS would very soon be solved."

Judith Lopez, San Francisco, CA

"I am an MD in clinical practice in Veracruz, Mexico. At the end of 1997, I gave an interview in *El Diario de Xalapa*, the most widely circulated newspaper in the state of Veracruz, stating that the causes of AIDS were not viral. As was expected, this created a great deal of controversy: most government officials immediately declared that my statements were wrong. At the same time, they refused all my invitations to debate the evidence upon which I based my statements.

"In response to my public challenges to the HIV hypothesis, I was contacted by several people diagnosed as HIV positive seeking alternative treatments for the conditions known as AIDS. The information I'd presented generated great doubt about the use of AZT and other antiretrovirals and protease inhibitors.

"I had been involved with the treatment of AIDS for over ten years. As the head of El Patronato Veracruzano de Lucha Contra el SIDA, I treated patients diagnosed with HIV that belonged to the lowest economic strata. Their inability to afford the drugs precluded me from giving them AZT, which has a high cost. As time went by, I began to see that the rich HIV positive patients died, while the poor ones lived and continue to do so. My questions about this situation were answered when my son, Alejandro Flores, sent me the book *Inventing the AIDS Virus* by Dr. Peter Duesberg.

"Using my new knowledge, so far I have treated 19 HIV positive and one HIV negative person, all of them males between the ages of 19 and 44. All patients suffered from malnutrition and belonged to the middle or lower economic class. Eight of these patients were treated with antiretrovirals such as AZT given to them by the state health agencies. During their antiretroviral treatment, they showed the typical symptoms: fever, weight loss, diarrhea, and pulmonary infections. They also suffered from depression due to the stigma of believing they had to die, enduring social ostracization and from unkind treatment by their families and others.

"The protocol that I gave them involved stopping the drug cocktails, antibiotics, antidepressants, anti-diarrheals and following a strict diet. Between two weeks and two months after beginning my protocol, the patients began to get better. Their symptoms began disappearing in this order: diarrhea, weight loss, pulmonary infections and depression.

"I would like to give a detailed account of two particular patients that I consider the most relevant. The first is a hair stylist, 33 years of age, homosexual, middle class, with a history of alcohol, cocaine and general drug abuse. He lived in constant conflict with his family because he was diagnosed with HIV in May of 1997. Upon being diagnosed, he began treatment in the AIDS clinic. In October of 1998, his family contacted me and asked to see me. I talked with the family on three occasions and on the third, I had the opportunity to meet with the patient himself. He had been taken to the hospital several times over the past year due to his delicate health condition. His last hospitalization was during the month of October. At that time, the doctors told him to go home and await his death among his family members. When we met, I explained my medical position and my clinical approach. He agreed to follow my treatment protocol without reservations. By the time we met, he had already lost 25 pounds, was immobilized in bed, and barely able to speak. When I said good-bye to him after our first meeting, he told me 'I know that I'm going to die.'

"The first week of treatment was very stressful for everybody, including myself. At the beginning of the second week the family of the patient began having serious doubts about the effectiveness of my protocol, but it was then that the patient started to show signs of improvement: first he began eating better, then his temperature returned to normal. Once he was able to get out of bed and sit in his rocking chair, he told me 'Doctor, I want to live.' By January 1999, he had gained 15 pounds while maintaining the diet that I prescribed, and returned to work.

"The second case is an HIV negative patient with the symptoms of full-blown AIDS. He is 25 years of age, single, and belongs to the upper middle class. In the last five years he has used antibiotics in high doses, mostly purchased over the counter and self-prescribed. In August of 1998, he started having symptoms that included pulmonary infections, frequent cough, and occasional diarrhea. By September, he began having fevers and was losing weight rapidly. He could not eat solid foods. He was hospitalized and his treatment consisted of more and more antibiotics. When I met him he told me 'I feel like I am going to die.' He was deeply anguished and depressed. His family thought that he had AIDS. They asked for my opinion and I told them that he was actually suffering a toxic immunodeficiency caused by the medicines given to him. Although he is HIV negative, I had him follow the exact same treatment given to my patients diagnosed with HIV. Needless to say, by January of 1999, all his symptoms were gone, he had gained close to 20 pounds and he was working again. His most recent HIV test is negative. These two cases are under total clinical control and are open to the scrutiny of those interested.

"In closing, I would like to let those people who suffer the stigma of an HIV positive diagnosis know that there are scientists that are willing to fight for the truth. You deserve to live."

Juan Jose Flores Rodriguez, MD, PhD, Veracruz, Mexico

If this book has altered your perspective on HIV and AIDS
or affected your life, please write or email us with the details.
We will send you a complimentary copy in exchange.
Your words may provide hope to others.

The American Foundation for AIDS Alternatives

Many experts now contend that AIDS is not a fatal, incurable condition caused by HIV, and that the symptoms associated with AIDS are treatable using nontoxic, immune-enhancing therapies that have restored the health of people diagnosed with AIDS and have allowed those at risk to remain well.

The American Foundation for AIDS Alternatives questions the HIV=AIDS=Death paradigm based on a growing body of scientific, medical, and epidemiological data and promotes awareness of life-affirming facts to HIV positive diagnosed persons and concerned citizens worldwide. We are a 501(c)3 nonprofit corporation founded by HIV positives who have learned to live in wellness without AIDS drugs and without fear of AIDS.

In addition to sponsoring medical research into practical, health-enhancing approaches to resolving AIDS and funding scientific studies that objectively examine the HIV hypothesis, we work locally by providing a yearly calendar of free community events and classes, and work globally by sharing our resources with other groups and associations throughout the world that promote informed choices for people affected by HIV and AIDS.

The American Foundation for AIDS Alternatives is one of the only AIDS organizations anywhere that does not solicit or accept funding from the pharmaceutical industry, the US government, or any entity that may limit public access to factual information about HIV, AIDS, and health.

The American Foundation for AIDS Alternatives
11684 Ventura Boulevard • Studio City, CA 91604
(877) 92-ALIVE • Email: AFAA@aliveandwell.org

Please send me ____ additional book(s) for $10.95 plus $2.00 postage per book.

❑ Enclosed is a check or money order ❑ Please bill my Visa or Mastercard

Cardholder Name ____________________

Account # ____________________ Expiration Date ____________

Signature ____________________

I want to support your efforts by including a tax-deductible donation:

❑ $25 ❑ $50 ❑ $100 ❑ $250 ❑ $500 ❑ $1000 ❑ $ ______

❑ Please send me a copy of your information catalog.

❑ Please add me to your national mailing list.

Name ____________________

Address ____________________

City ____________________ State ________ Zip ____________